Living Green with Smoothies and the Culture of Life

James C. Tibbetts

i

Disclaimer Notice: You have the constitutional right to prescribe for yourself and to determine your own diet and detoxification methods but the writers and publisher assume no responsibility. If you use the information in this book without the approval of a health professional, you prescribe for yourself, which remains your constitutional right. In addition while it would be inappropriate for the authors to steer individuals in decisions of omission or commission regarding therapies, it would be equally improper to shun responsibility of suggesting what we consider the best options for degenerative disease. The authors and publisher do not directly or indirectly dispense medical advice or prescribe the use of fasting or diet or other modality as a form of treatment for sickness without medical approval. Nutritionists and other health experts in the field of health and nutrition hold widely varying views. The authors and publisher do not intend to diagnose or prescribe.

The Scripture citations are taken in part or whole from various bibles including: *The New American Bible* (Thomas Nelson Publisher, 1970); *The Jerusalem Bible* (Doubleday & Co., 1966); *Revised Standard Version, Holy Bible from the Ancient Eastern Text*, translation from the *Aramaic of the Peshitta* by George M. Lamsa, (Harper San Francisco,1961).

Jim Tibbetts
P.O. Box 2533
Glenville, NY 12325

www.jimtibbetts.com

ISBN: 978-1-365-36724-3

Table of Contents

Table of Contents   iii
Introduction   vi

I.   Green Smoothies
     A. Planet Alleluia Green Zone   1
     B. Why Green Smoothies?   3
     C. Ann Wigmore and Blending   4
     D. The Importance of Taste   7

II. The Detox Healing Process
     A. Greens and Chlorophyll   8
     B. Detoxification   9
     C. Juice Fasting and Detoxification   12
     D. The Openshaw Green Smoothie Survey   17
     E. 21 Day Green Smoothie Detox program   21

III. Health and Healing with Chlorophyll
     A. Chlorophyll is Green Magic   24
     B. Wheatgrass, Concentrated Chlorophyll   26
     C. Healing with Chlorophyll   29
     D. Chlorophyll a Brief History   33
     E. What are Green Foods Supplements?   38

IV. Fiber and a Rainbow of Colors
     A. The Rainbow of Smoothie Colors   40
     B. Fiber in Smoothies   46
     C. Grains vs. Sprouted Grains   49
     D. Cooking Destroys Nutrients   53

V.   The Alkaline Body and Oxygen
     A. Alkaline Forming Foods   56
     B   Growing Fresh Air - Oxygen   63
     C. Green Tea   66

VI.   Green CAM Nutrition Therapy
    A. CAM and Green Paradigms   67
    B. Green Nutrition Therapy   72

VII. The Raw Family on Green Smoothies
    A. The Raw Family on Green Smoothies   77
    B. Ten Health Benefits, Green Smoothies   78
    C. Guidelines to Drinking, Smoothies   80
    D. Common Questions & Victoria   83
    E. Stomach Acid and Raw Foods   88
    F. The Roseburg Green Smoothie Study   91

VIII. Green Food Smoothie Creations
    A. Green Smoothie's   97
      a. Jim's Smoothies   99
      b. The Raw Family Green Smoothies   103
      c. 15 Green Smoothies in 3 Minutes   106
      d. Top Smoothie Ingredients liked?   108
      e. Several Raw Chefs Smoothies   111
    B. Smoothie Puddings   114
    C. Smoothie Soups
      a. Warming and Raw Soups   116
      b. Selected Raw Chefs Soups   120
    D. Salads and Salad Soups   125
    E. Patés and Paté Short Soups   128

IX.   Spiritual Nutrition
    A. Purification of the Body   134
    B. Fasting and Healing   136
    C. Kosher, Pure Foods   137
    D. A Toxicology Study on the Torah   140
    E. Early Writers on the Essenes   143
    F. Christianity a Continuation- Essenes   146
    G. James the Second Pope was Vegetarian   148
    H. Essene Community- New Covenant   149

    I.   First Jewish-Christian Communities
           Considered Jesus a Vegetarian   152
    J. Those seeking the Culture of Life   156
    K. Purification and Consecration   160

IX. Resources
    A. Raw Vegan Uncook books   165
    B. Green Powders   168
    C. Plant-based Protein Powders   169

X. Appendix
    A. Bio - Jim Tibbetts   176
    B. Endnotes   178

Introduction

This work is a review of the literature of chlorophyll rich foods especially smoothies. Dr. Ann Wigmore, Victoria Boutenko and other well known names in this field are written about. A brief historical review and scientific review of chlorophyll is presented. Several surveys of the benefits of green smoothies are incorporated and healing aspects of chlorophyll are included. Many of the key concepts and teachings of chlorophyll are found in the chapters. In addition the practical side of eating chlorophyll rich foods as smoothies and smoothie soups is presented with many receipts from various chefs.

This book is cutting edge science on the topic of chlorophyll rich foods such as green juices and smoothies, salads and soups. Cutting edge science points in a certain direction from a limited amount of data and research. But this is where scientific discoveries start by heading in a certain direction. This book is well documented showing a solid scientific foundation to build upon.

The revolution of using Chlorophyll rich foods such as green smoothies and green soups for optimum health and healing is well underway for over half a century. The raw foods and Living Foods movements are being used to heal many major degenerative diseases, and chlorophyll rich foods are found to be at the center of nearly all of these healings.

In the chapter on "Chlorophyll a Brief History" is research that is foundational to this book: "Many of these blood-building components are found in chlorophyll rich foods such as cereal glasses (wheat, oats, barley, etc.) and dark green vegetables. Young cereal plants absorb and synthesize vitamin K, vitamin C, folic acid, pyridoxine, iron, calcium and protein for their growth and development. These very same nutrients are essential to the generation and utilization of hemoglobin in humans and animals."[1]

As far back as 1926 journal research suggested a relationship between the chlorophyll and hemoglobin generation.[2] Journal studies in 1933 indicated that feeding chlorophyll-rich foods to rats triggered the regeneration of red blood cells.[3] In 1934, a journal study discovered that chlorophyll stimulated the synthesis of red blood cells in a variety of animals.[4] This was the beginning of a serious scientific interest in chlorophyll rich foods.

Both the practical side of making smoothies, soups, pates, salads and juices are written about in this work but also the scientific and historical aspects of chlorophyll rich foods. It is the relationship between human blood and chlorophyll that brings a lot of the curing capabilities found in Greens!

The whole point of this lifestyle is the focus on Living Foods and not dead foods; this is a diet, a nutritional program that is based on the Culture of Life and not the Culture of Death and degenerative disease. This is why the chapter on Spiritual Nutrition was added which shows the biblical and spiritual reasons why this type of nutritional lifestyle is important and has biblical and spiritual roots. This chapter is more along the lines of professional theology showing the solid biblical and theological evidence. This section is an edit from my book showing that Jesus Christ was a vegetarian along with a lot of his disciples.

For many years I used to promote a plant-based diet to people now I focus on this book since getting them interested in this lifestyle and allowing their body to progress at its own rate. It is important to start moving in this direction and as the body's parameters change (pH, sodium-potassium levels, other levels) and become normal and optimal their diet will adjust itself, if the person listens to their body.

I hope that this book helps you to move forward in staying healthy and in healing whatever health condition that you need to address, through green smoothies and other chlorophyll rich foods.

The last section on Spiritual Nutrition gives a condensed insight into the early Church and their emphasis on food in community and for life.

"My dear friend, I hope you are in good health and may you thrive in all other ways as you do in the spirit." 3 John 2

To your health and healing in Christ
Jim Tibbetts

Chapter I
Green Smoothies

A. Planet Alleluia Green Zone

One of the greatest therapies for health and healing illnesses and degenerative diseases is to enter the Green Zone and shout Alleluia. There are three main types of plant-based diets: vegetarian, vegan and raw vegan. On the plant-based diets such as a raw vegan or Living Foods diet you eat a lot of produce, especially greens and after a while a person desires greens, and salads and vegetables. For degenerative diseases, a person needs to nutritionally enter into and stay in the, Alleluia Green Zone!

Thus it is recommended that at least one or two or three of these every day is needed to help achieve and remain in the Green Zone in nutrition.
- A green smoothie
- Green superfoods
- A shot of wheat grass or barley grass
- A glass or several glasses of green juice
- A large salad with Kale and/or other greens

This recommendation is not just from research and experience but from the experience and recommendations of other experts in the field. These suggestions are found in plant based diets such as:

- Gerson Diet: several glasses of green juice
    (Max Gerson, MD)
- Hippocrates Diet: raw greens, wheat grass daily
    (Anne Wigmore, PhD, Brian Clements, PhD
        and following)
- The pH miracle Diet: Super Greens every day.
    (Robert Young, PhD)

- Rainbow Green Diet: Kale and other greens daily
    (Gabriel Cousens, MD)
- Sunfood Diet: many green superfoods
    (David Wolfe, MS)
- Raw Family Diet: a large green smoothie daily
    (Victoria, Valya and Sergei Boutenko)
- Raw Revolution Diet: many greens in general
    (Cherie Soria, Brenda Davis, RD and
      Vesanto Melina, MS, RD)
- Alleluia Diet: several green foods every day
    (Jim Tibbetts, STL, MBA)
- Hallelujah Diet: barley grass and blended green foods
    (Rev. George Malkamus, DD)
- Natural Hygiene Diet: lots of greens every day
    (Greg Haag, MD and Tosca Haag, MD and others)
- The Healthy Journey Diet, lots of greens
    (Fred Bisci, PhD)

For those in the raw food field many of these names will be recognized and many more could be added. The important thing is the constant refrain of "Greens" and "Chlorophyll Rich Foods".

One reason for this apparent need is the closeness of the chlorophyll molecule to blood. Greens supply us with chlorophyll. Chlorophyll's molecular structured is very similar to the hemoglobin molecule of blood. The molecular structures of human blood and of chlorophyll are identical except that human blood has iron as its center and chlorophyll has magnesium at its center. This has many benefits that have been documented over the decades and some are reported in this book.

Cooking and heating can destroy the chlorophyll in foods, which is why raw foods are best. The following chapter on cooking will explain this further.

B. Why Green Smoothies?

Green smoothies are one of the easiest, most delicious and fun ways to get greens into your diet. People with degenerative diseases need even more green foods in their diet, because the chlorophyll is a blood purifier and has many notable activities in the body and therapeutic activity. To eat the amount of greens that is needed is difficult. Green food powders are one way to get around this and have become very popular and successful. Also the blender opens up the plant cells to let the chlorophyll and nutrients out to get into your system easier.

By taking a salad and putting it into a high powered blender[1] and blending it a person can consume several times the amount of vegetables that used to be consumed by chewing. Blending the salads increases considerably the cell building nutrients and fiber.

Green smoothies are basically a blend of green vegetables and fruits and other stuff. There are many variations. A basic one that I use is to start with a banana and water or juice and blend it, add some lettuce blend it, add another fruit or vegetable or two blend it, add some protein powder, flax seed oil and some green powder blend it, add whatever else I want and blend it. It can be a whole meal in one glass!

The benefit of green smoothies is not only in the extremely healthy mixture just mentioned above, but that it gives a place to add many of your nutrient supplements to in a tasty way. Add some of the daily nutrients, flax oil and protein powder that you'll have to take, into the green smoothie and blend it up, than drink it down!

---

[1] Like a *Vita Mix* or *Health Master* or other blender

Green smoothies, wheatgrass or other freshly juiced greens, keep the greens in their colloidal form which is closest to the human body. This is the highest form of taking in chlorophyll, trace minerals, phytonutrients and other essentials in greens. Powdered greens come in a close second to the value of fresh greens.

C. Ann Wigmore and Blending

Ann Wigmore is one of the founders of the living foods movement. Her teachings on sprouting and wheatgrass have put these in almost every health food store and many supermarkets across the country. Back in the 1960's she worked at solving her personal health problems through living foods and then started helping others by teaching them a living foods program. She wrote some books on her efforts and one of them, *The Blending Book, Maximizing Nature's Nutrients*, (1970's) she writes on the benefits of blending foods and a diet with a lot of blended foods. The following are a few key paragraphs from this book to show her teachings and emphasis.

"The living foods lifestyle is more than just a diet; it is a way of taking total responsibility for your nutritional needs. Living foods are the most nutritious foods that exist, and they are all offered in an easy-to-digest form. Living foods include super-nutritious young organic greens; power-packed sprouted nuts, seeds, and grains; and fabulous fermented preparations. In addition, fresh wheatgrass juice adds an unparalleled level of nutritional healing and vitality. All of these foods are prepared without cooking, since cooking destroys the life force in the enzymes. The living foods lifestyle uses no meat, dairy foods, or other animal products."[5]

4

"Perhaps the question most frequently asked by those beginning to practice the living foods lifestyle is, 'Why blend practically everything that is eaten?' The answer is simple. Blending is the easiest and most efficient way to provide food that is both nourishing and easy to digest. By blending foods, we can counteract the poor eating habits most of us have developed over the years, and that are the cause of many of the physical problems we have."[6]

"If you are healthy, blending will help you to stay that way. Blended living foods are full of vitamins, minerals, enzymes, and other nutrients, and since they are easy to digest and assimilate, they give your body more of what it needs to keep functioning at top condition. The most important key to health is to use blended foods in small amounts frequently throughout the day. I realize that this may seem drastic, but if you are serious about maintaining or restoring your health, I can assure you that this is the most beneficial way. And remember, the living foods lifestyle is a guide for the highest level of health, in which the body is free of illnesses and full of energy.

I have seen so many students come to my centers with all kinds of diseases. There is absolutely no doubt in my mind that every one of these people suffers from an inability to assimilate nourishment, which leads to deficiencies and illnesses. When easy-to-digest, high-energy blended foods are provided, the changes in their health are immediate. Unfortunately, in our society, unhealthy eating habits, and therefore illnesses, tend to prevail.

In our society, we tend to eat food in chunks, swallowing it quickly after very little chewing. This means that the enzymes in the mouth do not have a chance to start the digestive process by breaking down the starch content of our food. As a result, as the food progresses through the digestive tract, it is inadequately prepared for assimilation. This, in turn, means that much of the nutrition the food should provide is not absorbed, and is eventually excreted as waste. Years of poor eating habits are likely to have an adverse effect on the entire system by physiologically altering its structure; a person with a poor digestive system will not have a healthy, balanced body."[7]

Anne Wigmore continues, "We have all known people who, through they eat enormous amounts of food, remain undernourished and are never completely healthy. This is because their digestive systems are faulty, and they do not benefit from the nutrition in the food they eat. An unhealthy diet leads to a digestive system that can't function properly. Living foods have been developed so that even the most severe digestive problems can be overcome through easy-to-digest, high-energy nourishment. Every food allows your body to receive optimal nutrition.

Blending the right types of food means that the body will have a chance to recover from those years of abuse or neglect, and, while it recovers, it will be relieved of the extra effort required to digest and assimilate, but solid foods, such as easy-to-chew uncooked vegetables, cannot be avoided, because the body needs a certain amount of fiber for elimination. My personal opinion is that a diet should consist of 70 percent blended foods and 30 percent other living foods. But each person has a different system and different needs; one must learn to listen to his or her own body."[8]

In the conclusion: "I hope that you will recognize that the body always has been and always will be a self-healer. It cannot fail if you work with nature, rather than against it. There is an incredible need for all of us to become interested in the tools of nature. When we use blended live foods in a balanced diet, we not only balance our own lives, but we become able to balance our planet. Through your own efforts, you will gain confidence that your body's capabilities will provide the needed results, enabling you to accomplish what you want to accomplish in your lifetime. As you connect with nature, you are connecting with your higher self."[9]

D. The Importance of Taste

Is taste important? Yes it is yet sometimes things do not taste good but are good for you. But taste can tell you if something has gone bad or rancid. Taste has an important part to play but it needs to evolve.

In the beginning stages most people's taste buds are conditioned to acidic foods and acidic tastes, sweet foods and unnatural sweet taste, salty, spicy foods and unnatural salty and spicy taste. A transition takes place in the taste buds when going from the unhealthy, unnatural standard American diet lifestyle to a healthy vegetarian, raw vegan lifestyle. One of the reasons for this is that acidic foods condition the taste to like acidic foods, which is bad. Alkaline foods allow the body's natural pH to take control and the taste buds become more alkaline, their natural state. Then eating a lot of greens and chlorophyll foods taste better naturally.

Should smoothies and chlorophyll rich foods taste good? Again, yes it is important and no it is not important. If you have a lot of green vegetables in your smoothies it is not going to be sweet, like smoothies that have a lot of fruit. In the beginning stages it is helpful that the smoothies and blended foods taste good to get them involved but after months the taste buds will readjust and all the sweet fruits and honey and other sweeteners in the smoothies will not be needed. Your taste buds will adapt and what tasted harsh weeks before will taste better. But in the long run yes, you want it to taste good too.

Chapter II
The Detox Healing Process

A. Greens and Chlorophyll

Victoria Boutenko could be called the Queen of the Green Smoothie revolution, she writes about some of the benefits of chlorophyll: "Chlorophyll has been proven helpful in preventing and healing many forms of cancer and arteriosclerosis. Chlorophyll: Builds a high blood count; helps prevent cancer; provides iron to organs; makes the body more alkaline; counteracts toxins eaten; improves anemic conditions; cleans and deodorizes bowel tissues; helps purify the liver; aids hepatitis improvement; regulates menstruation; aids hemophilia condition; helps sores heal faster; eliminates body odors; resists bacteria in wounds; cleans tooth and gum structure in pyorrhea; eliminates bad breath."[10]

Victoria makes a good point about mixing starches and fruits. "Many nutritionists believe, starchy tubers combined in one meal with sour fruits or vegetables can create fermentation and gas in our intestines. Placing greens in the same category as vegetables has caused people to mistakenly apply the combining rules of starchy vegetables to greens. Driven by this confusion, many concerned people wrote to me inquiring if blending fruits with greens was proper food combining. They had heard that 'fruits and vegetables did not mix well.' Yes, to combine starchy vegetables with fruits would not be a good idea. Such a combination can cause gas in the intestines. However, greens are not vegetables and greens are not starchy. In fact, greens are the only food group that helps digest other foods through stimulating the secretion of digestive enzymes. Thus, greens can be combined with any other foods."[11]

8

Dr. Benjamin Gurskin, the past director of experimental pathology at Temple University, was published in the *American Journal of Surgery*. Dr. Gurskin discussed more than one thousand cases in which various disorders were treated with chlorophyll. Commenting on his associates' experiences with chlorophyll, he wrote, "It is interesting to note that there is not a single case recorded in which either improvement or cure has not taken place."[12]

B. Detoxification

Detoxification is a step by step process, an easy way to understand detoxification is by understanding three layers of tubes in the body. The first layer is the digestive system which goes from the stomach to the intestines to the colon. The second layer is the circulatory system which includes the arteries, veins, capillaries, and heart. The third layer is the lymphatic system which surrounds and bathes all the organs, muscles, and all the body's tissues and cells.

The blood stream draws the nourishment from the digestive system and the lymphatic system draws nourishment from the blood stream to feed the cells. Then the lymphatic system delivers the cells' waste products back to the blood, which delivers the waste to the colon for disposal.

Of course it is a bit more complicated than just three tubes passing nutrients there are other organs, such as the liver, which are also involved. But the process is the same whether it is food or smoothies or juices yet they have distinct differences. By eating dense foods, especially cooked foods, a person increases the density of the body's tube fluids, especially the lymph fluids, which can cause congestion of the system. This can cause a dampening effect on the electrical nervous system which disrupts or deadens the neural transmissions, giving a dulling of the senses or tiredness or sleepiness. Most people experience this on a heavy meal.

For juices, smoothies and other food that is light, nutritious and primarily living foods, those filled with life, this sense of dullness, heaviness, tired or sleepiness may not be there. More importantly the blood is not just a carrier but also nourished and filled with more energy (on the microscopic level). When this gets to the lymph system it also has more energy which it receives from the blood stream, it is less congested and more alive with more nutrients for itself (bio-chemically) and for the organs it is delivering the foods and nourishment too.

With smoothies and also juices this can become detoxifying and the cellular system can then release toxins, poisons, unused or poor quality food nourishment back into the lymph system for waste removal. Thus the good pushes out the bad. This sometimes brings a detox backlash since a person may get headaches, gas, intestinal discomfort, nausea, rashes, etc. as the 'bad' is released and replaced by the 'good'. These cleansing symptoms are common and usually short lived. These bad chemicals in the body often cause negative impulses and unnatural desires, which also are purged from the system.

Numerous scientific studies have been done showing the chemicals and poisons in the food chain. "During the past three decades, surveillance of toxic exposure in the U.S. population has been a routine governmental practice. Since 1970, for example, the U.S. Environmental Protection Agency (EPA) has conducted the National Human Adipose Tissue Survey (NHATS) to determine the prevalence of fat-soluble toxins in the fat cells in U.S. citizens.[13] The 1986 version of this survey, for example, analyzed 671 adipose tissue specimens to determine the prevalence of 111 toxic compounds."[14]

Studies on tissues and body fluids and bone show the presence of numerous toxins in the body, including toxins that could be in the food or the environment: DDE & DDT &, B-BHC,[15] TCDD,[16] p-DCB,[17] Lead,[18] Mercury,[19] Cadmium,[20] PBBs,[21] 2,5-DCP & l-naphthol & 3,5,6-TCP & 2-naphthol & 3,5,6-TCP & PCP, 4-nitrophenol, (pesticide residues in urine in adults in U.S.)[22] Styrene & Vinyl chloride (packaging migrant),[23] Toluene (Solvent),[24] Xylene (solvent)[25].

And there are also toxins directly related to or in the foods: Acetone (pesticide solvent),[26] Arsenic (arsenical pesticides),[27] Benzene (solvent for pesticide formulations),[28] Bromobenzene (fumigant precursor),[29] Carbon tetrachloride (former fumigant),[30] Ethylene dibromide (fumigant),[31] Ethylene dichloride (fumigant),[32] Hexane (solvent),[33] Kepone (pesticide),[34] Methoxychlor (insecticide),[35] Methy isobutyl ketone (synthetic flavoring),[36] Methylene chloride (decaffeinator),[37] and studies on coal tar dye colorings containing polycyclic aromatic hydrocarbons.[38]

The use of chemicals in foods has soared from 419 million pounds in 1955 to more than 800 million today (1968). Each of us eats more than three pounds of food additives a year.[39] Added to the intentional and unintentional chemicals in our foods are the chemicals we ingest as medicines. Americans are the most medicated people in the world. Every year we swallow 37 billion doses of therapeutic pills, powders, capsules, and elixirs.[40] No one knows what effect the combinations of pesticides, food additives; and medicines may have. (These figures of 419 lbs. to 800 pounds or 37 billion doses of pills were cited from the late 1960's and would obviously be more today.)

In addition to the foods we eat and the medicines we take, we fill the sky with over 130 tons of noxious chemicals... carbon monoxides, hydrocarbons, nitrogen oxides, sulfur oxides, and particulates. Persons living in New York may inhale the equivalent of 730 pounds of chemicals a year. Just think you astronauts are the average America who has all these poisons and chemicals in you bodies! A person needs to eat raw living foods and go on long fasts and get rid of all this garbage.

Most medical professionals and scientists don't think in terms of poisons, toxins, pollutants and parasites but the best way to deal with these is fasting and a raw vegan diet. What is the difference between poisons and toxins? Poisons generally come from outside the body as just described above. Toxins are produced from within the body by various means usually parasites.

Gabriel Cousens, MD (citing the research of Robert Young, PhD) points out that: "A typical modern-day meal featuring a main course of beef, poultry, or fish may contain up to 750 million pathogenic microorganisms per servings, compared to a typical vegan meal containing only 500 pathogenic microorganisms per meal."[41] So the problem is not just inorganic poisons and pollutants but also living bad microorganisms.

C. Juice Fasting and Detoxification

Both drinking juices and smoothies are means of detoxification and a means of resetting the biochemistry to optimize it. Fasting is one of the major means of detoxification and some of the concepts and principles are the same or very similar. In the author's book; *Juice Fasting Simplified a Practical Approach*. Fasting does various things to bring health and healing to the body the two main ones are: detoxification and resetting the biochemistry. Everyone knows that fasting is a detoxification method but most people don't know that on a long fast the biochemistry of the body gets reset (little by little) back to its normal perfect operating mode. On a long fast the biochemistry is reset and healing starts taking place since the body becomes optimized and starts to heal itself.

The food we eat goes through several stages; first it is chewed, masticated; then digested and assimilated; and finally eliminated as waste. The four main organs of elimination are the bowels, the kidneys, the lungs and the skin. A meal goes from the mouth through a thirty-foot tube known as the gastrointestinal tract to the rectum. Liquid passes through about two million filtering fibers in the human kidneys. The body with all its organs works harmoniously through these stages to bring nutrition to the billions of body cells.

The bowels eliminate two things; food wastes and body waste. Food waste is from the food we eat. The body waste is from the blood and tissues which are discharged into the intestinal canal and in the bowels, these body wastes are excreted from the body. If the body waste is not eliminated, it would cause protein petrifaction resulting in toxemia or acidosis. The kidneys excrete the end products of food and body metabolism from the liver. Perspiration throws off toxins through the sweat glands. The lungs give off carbon dioxide and possibly other gases. This internal elimination is accelerated during the fasting process.

The process of autolysis or self-digestion occurs during a fast. During the first few days, the body will live on its own fast and stored substances. After this is depleted, the body starts to burn and digest its own tissues. The body first burns up the cells which are dead, aged, damaged and diseased tissues, tumors, fat deposits, etc. Fasting gets rid of the inferior cells and keeps the essential ones.

Fasting is not starving. Starving is the process of dying. When a person does not eat, the body enters into a fasting period. This second period can go on for weeks or even a month or two. This third period that a person's body enters into is the stage of starvation. The fasting stage continues as long as the body has stored reserves in the tissues. During this fasting stage, the body continues to nourish itself just as if it were eating. And detoxification also occurs at this time.

When the fasting stage is over with, genuine hunger is experienced. The hunger pains in the beginning of a fast are normal gastric contractions or stomach spasms. These are merely the sensation of hunger and not true hunger. This false hunger is normal for the first few days of a fast.

The cells in our body exist in three stages; new developing cells, fully developed cells and old dying cells needing to be replaced. Waste products in the cells interfere with the nourishment of the cells. These older dying cells and poisoned cells need to be flushed out of our bodies. *By fasting, these cells with the mucus, toxins and poisons will be flushed out of the body through the kidneys.*

The question may arise, **what poisons in my body**? Many books have been written to answer that question. Today there are many chemicals that have toxic effects on the body. These can come from prescription drugs, cleaning compounds, kitchen detergents, garden insecticides and industrial chemicals. A few of the common poisons are: Carbon monoxide from air pollution; DDT and other pesticides sprayed on foods; mercury; lead from gasoline, paint and other industrial sources; ozone, nitrogen dioxide and cadmium are air pollutants coming from smog; wax sprayed on fruits and vegetables to give a longer shelf life and makes them look better; most food colorings are synthetic and coal-tar based; artificial flavorings are either natural or synthetic and comprise about two thirds of all food additives used in America. And irradiation kills the enzymes not just bacteria and germs. The previous section went through a long list of these.

Fasting is one of the best ways to get rid of poisons, toxins, pesticides, waxes and other synthetic chemicals that can be found in fruits and vegetables. Fasting catabolizes the dead, diseased and pesticide ridden cells and flushes them out of the body. Fasting is the best way to get rid of pesticides. Thus there is a simple and universal answer to this major worldwide problem. The answer is fasting! Fasting is one of the best methods of ridding the body of commercial poisons and toxins. Fasting is a simple, inexpensive way to insure health and happiness.

Green smoothies and green drinks are also a major way of detoxification of these poisons, toxins, pesticides and other chemicals from the body. The properties of these are found in other chapters.

Clean inside means eating foods which flow through us, leaving their amino acid proteins, enzymes, minerals, vitamins, and other vital energies. This food should not stop to putrefy and ferment. Clean inside means having a good acid-alkaline balance in the digestive system, a balance which avoids acid-caused toxic conditions throughout the body. Clean inside means a well-working bloodstream will supplied with health promoting minerals and having a liver capable of detoxifying the impurities which run through it.

Furthermore, there are reasons for our ill health and that we are toxic; 1. Environmental poisons and toxins and drugs (coming from outside in); 2. Toxins built up within out body on a cellular level (toxins being created on the inside); and 3. Parasites and worms within us, (which also give off toxic wastes). Fasting may or may not kill all of them.

Juice fasting involves drinking fruit and vegetable juices, vegetables and herbal teas. These are easily assimilated into the upper digestive tract and do not stimulate the secretion of hydrochloric acid in the stomach.

The question has been asked if juice fasting is a real fast or just a liquid diet? Dr. Airola responds, "Any condition when your body is encouraged to initiate the process of autolysis, or self-digestion, is fasting. During juice fasting, when no solid foods, proteins or fats are consumed, your body will decompose and burn all the diseased and inferior protein and fat tissues, just as it does during the water fast. Juices are absorbed directly into the bloodstream without the usual process of digestion."[42]

Dr. Airola presents a list of scientific justifications for juice fasting which he bases on physiological facts and professional opinions:

1. Raw Juices and broths "are rich in vitamins, minerals, trace elements and enzymes."

2. "These vital elements are very easily assimilated directly into the bloodstream, without putting a strain on the digestive system - thus they do not disrupt the healing and rejuvenating process of autolysis, or self-digestion."

3. Juices "do not stimulate the secretion of hydrochloric acid in the stomach."

4. "The nutritive elements from the juices are extremely beneficial in normalizing all the body processes, supplying needed elements for the body's own healing activity and cell regeneration, and, thus, speeding the recovery."

5. "Raw juices and vegetable broths provide an alkaline surplus which is extremely important for the proper acid-alkaline balance in the blood and tissues, since blood and tissues contain large amounts of acids during fasting."

6. "Generous amounts of minerals in the juices, particularly in the vegetable broth, help to restore the biochemical and mineral balance in the tissues and cells."

7. Numerous fasting clinics and experts make scientific claims as well:

a) "According to Dr. Ralph Bircher, raw juices contain an as yet unidentified factor which stimulates what he calls a micro-electric tension in the body and is responsible for the cells' ability to absorb nutrients from the blood stream and effectively excrete metabolic wastes."

b) Dr. Ragnar Berg a leading authority on nutrition and biochemistry states; "During fasting the body burns up and excretes huge amounts of accumulated wastes. We can help this cleansing process by drinking alkaline juices instead of water while fasting. I have supervised may fasts and made extensive tests of fasting patients, and I am convinced that drinking alkaline-forming fruit and vegetable juices, instead of water, during fasting will increase the healing effect of fasting. Elimination of uric acid and other inorganic acids will be accelerated. And sugars in juices will strengthen the heart...Juice fasting is, therefore, the best form of fasting."

c) Dr. Otto H.F. Buchinger at his clinic has supervised over 80,000 fasts and employs only juice fasting. "He told me that, in his experience, fasting on the fresh raw juices of fruits and vegetables, plus vegetable broths and herb teas, results in much faster recover from disease and more effective cleansing and rejuvenation of the tissues that does the traditional water fast."[43]

Drinking juices allows for the body to assimilate all of the vital substances in the quickest possible time. It may only take ten to fifteen minutes to assimilate juices properly made. But it may take several hours to digest juice that is still in the pulp or liquefied stage (with solids). Juices give the cells in the body all the elements they need in a way that is easily assimilated.

D. The Openshaw Green Smoothie Survey

Many others have jumped on the bandwagon to promote green smoothies since Victoria Boutenko started the green smoothie revolution. The following study helps to further strengthen the argument of the benefits of green smoothies.

In the book; *The Green Smoothies Diet, the Natural Program for Extraordinary Health* by Robyn Openshaw[44] she did a survey/study on green smoothies.[45] She collected the data from 175 respondents who had been drinking green smoothies for at least 30 days. This is an excellent example of the benefits of drinking green smoothies.

Research Results

"The results of my poll of 175 green-smoothie drinkers yielded some interesting results that suggest quite definitively that it's a ten-minute habit worth adopting! To participate in the questionnaire, one had to be drinking green smoothies for at least 30 days, a pint a day for at least three days a week. Many were drinking more, then to my recommended quart daily.

The vast majority, or 95.4 percent, said green smoothies noticeably improved their health or quality of life. Very exciting to me is the fact that 84 percent of those drinking green smoothies are so enthusiastic about the positive health benefits that they've told others about or taught them the habit!

These are the positive health effects people experience, listed in order of their frequency among the research respondents:
- 85 percent experience more energy.
- 79.5 percent experience improved digestion (more regular and/or complete bowel movements, no straining, soft/formed stool, etc.)
- 65 percent experience fewer cravings for sweets and processed foods.
- 54 percent experience a more positive, stable mood.
- 50 percent experience an improvement in skin tone, or fewer blemishes.
- 50 percent experience weight loss. The average reported pounds lost were 18.25 pounds!

(Keep in mind when considering this very impressive statistic that some of the respondents had been drinking green smoothies only 30 days, and some of them did not have any weight to lose. But 87 out of 175 respondents reported a total of over 15-- 0 pounds of weight lost!)

- 46.3 percent experience an increased desire to exercise.
- 45 percent experience improved sleep (need less of it, decreased insomnia, more alert in the mornings, etc.).
- 44 percent feel less stressed out.
- 39 percent experience blood sugar stabilization.
- 37 percent say their fingernails are stronger or grow faster.
- 36 percent experience people telling them they look better.
- 27.5 percent say their hair is shinier or their dandruff gone.
- 22 percent experience a decrease in PMS symptoms. (Consider that some of the respondents in the survey are not females of menstruating age).
- 20 percent report an improved sex drive.

Other positive health benefits reported by survey respondents include:
- 8 people said: Arthritis symptoms/pain gone or reduced
- 3 people said: Hyperthyroid condition improved (reduced or gone off meds)
- 2 people said: Seasonal allergies gone or decreased
- 3 people said: Reduced asthma symptoms
- 2 people said: Migraines gone or reduced by 80 percent
- 2 people said: Acne improved or gone
- 2 people said: Eczema or dry skin cleared
- 2 people said: Gray hair returned to original color
- 2 people said: Gallstones gone
- 2 people said: Decreased blood pressure
- No more hypertension
- Was able to go off cholesterol meds
- Was able to go off Prilosec
- Haven't gotten sick in a year like I always do

- Moles disappeared
- Deep facial wrinkles "barely noticeable"
- Less nasal congestion
- Lump or leg getting smaller
- Live spots fading
- Tendonitis gone
- Muscle soreness gone
- Fibromyalgia symptoms disappearing
- Hypoglycemia improved
- No more bloating, gas, indigestion, constipation
- Avoided a hysterectomy
- 2 people said lifelong menstrual problems returned to normal
- Hot flashes stopped
- No more aching muscles after hard workouts
- No more reflux/nausea after eating
- No more insomnia
- Easier to breastfeed
- Don't sunburn anymore
- Depression symptoms gone
- Lifelong bad breath gone in two weeks
- Ended coffee addition
- More alkaline body pH
- Just feel better

Only 18.3 percent had uncomfortable, short-term cleansing reactions. The following symptoms were reported:

Headaches	Dizziness
Diarrhea	Lethargy or weakness
Bloating	Runny nose
Cramps	Cold/virus
Vertigo	Depression
Fainting	Mucus in the back of throat
Skin breakouts	Liver pain/liver cleansing
Nausea	Mood swings
Intestinal gas	Emotional crisis
Constipation	

The risks of a new green-smoothie habit are limited to an 18.3 percent chance of short-term discomfort. The top six benefits that people experience when starting a green smoothie habit are, in order:
- more energy,
- improved digestion,
- fewer cravings for sweets and processed food,
- a more positive/stable mood,
- improved skin,
- and weight loss."[46]

Long term benefits are not in the survey, but long term benefits would include remission and healing from various illnesses and perhaps even from some degenerative diseases (when combined with a Living Foods diet).

E. 21 Day Green Smoothie Detox program

Many people today need a program to get started to detox their bodies. Along with the body there is the roller-coaster of emotions and foods, thinking patterns on eating, cultural and personal dietary habits, interpersonal relationships connected to foods, misunderstood theories or philosophies about diets, decades of mis-information about diets and detox. All of this can make the detox process more difficult. A simple way to do it is a Green Smoothie Detox!

We all have a physiological body, a psychological soul and a human spirit. The human spirit is really a different paradigm, a different dimension from the body-soul dimension which is within space-time-energy causality continuum, in the world of science. This book doesn't get into the spiritual dimension in the world of theology. Let us simply say the human spirit is uplifted and brightened during fasting and detox methods, yes even through a green smoothie detox. A detox of the body also means you are also working with detoxing the soul, the psychological. The two are closely tied together.

Increasing the level and intensity of greens in the diet is what it is all about; this increases the chlorophyll in the body and all the healing aspects that go along with it. It is a growing experience to get more and more greens into your diet. After a while people start getting excited about things like Kale! There is actually an increase in the desire for greens; we develop a love for "Greens"!

Some people recommend a 7 day or a 14 day detox program and these are good but the standard juice fast in European fasting clinics is a 21 to a 28 day juice fast. The detoxification in fasting starts in the 3rd day and a minor detox happens within 7 days. It takes about 14 days to enter into the next level where therapeutic fasting begins, by 21 days the healing process has had enough time to do a major detox in the body. So the goal is to shoot for 21 days.

21 Day Green Smoothie Detox program

1st week
1 to 2 Green smoothies every day
1 to 2 glasses of fresh juice every day
3 day transition to a plant-based diet

2nd week
2 to 3 green smoothies every day
2 to 3 glasses of fresh juice every day
Large salad at either lunch or dinner which is the main meal
The other meal is 80/20 raw vegan. Breakfast can be just smoothies and juices.

3rd week
3 to 5 green smoothies every day
3 to 7 glasses of juice every day
4 to 7 days of complete green smoothies

During the 21 day smoothie detox diet, you can drink all the water you want but avoid carbonated beverages, alcohol, and other unhealthy drinks!

The first week can be a lacto-ovo-vegetarian diet, moving away from most all animal products and most processed foods and drinks. The second week it is best to move into a strict vegan or raw vegan diet, away from all animal products and all grain products and most if not all cooking. Don't worry about the protein; mix a scoop of vegan protein powder in with your smoothie if you think you need it. The second week, get off all animal and grain products and all processed food products if possible. The third week is a raw vegan diet with smoothies.

By the third week when you are just drinking juices and smoothies it is very close to juice fasting. The process of juice fasting involves no solids and only juices but this is about as close to a juice fast as you can get. Autolysis starts happening in a juice fast where the dead, diseased and dying cells start to get flushed out of the body. This third week is very close to juice fasting and thus this process may start happening on a deeper level. See the author's juice fasting book, *Juice Fasting Simplified a Practical Approach* for a detailed explanation.

After 21 days just start moving back into eating normal. Take 2 to 3 days to moving back into a healthy diet which is primarily plant-based if not totally.

Chapter III

Health and Healing with Chlorophyll

"The body heals itself. The patient is only Nature's
assistant."   Greek physician Hippocrates

A. Chlorophyll is Green Magic

Brian Clements, PhD (involved in this field since the
1970's) in his book: *Living Foods for Optimum Health*,[47] has
some good comments: "You know that all life requires
oxygen, but you may not know that the foods we eat can rob
that life-giving oxygen from our cells, causing disease and
death. That's why it's important to be sure that we select
foods that feed, rather than rob, oxygen. But how can we
know which foods give and which foods take oxygen?

"If you recall your early science lesson about
photosynthesis, you'll remember that all plants, terrestrial
and aquatic, absorb water and carbon dioxide and then give
off oxygen as a waste product. That's why botanical food is
composed of oxygen in the molecular structure of its
chlorophyll content. Chlorophyll is the 'blood' of a plant. It
is the protein in plant life that gives it its distinctive green or
purple color. When compared to a molecule of hemoglobin
(the oxygen carrier in human blood) chlorophyll is almost
identical. Have you ever thought about what happens to that
oxygen when we eat those foods in their living state? It feeds
oxygen to our body - the oxygen we need to stay alive and
healthy. Only living foods bring that oxygen into the body.

"The value of chlorophyll isn't a new discovery. In
the early part of the twentieth century, chlorophyll was
regarded as a top-notch weapon in the arsenal of
pharmacopoeia. Many physicians used it as a treatment for

various complaints such as ulcers and skin disease, and as a pain reliever and breath freshener. One report by Dr. Benjamin Gurskin, then director of experimental pathology at Temple University, was published in the *American Journal of Surgery*. Dr. Gurskin discussed more than one thousand cases in which various disorders were treated with chlorophyll. Commenting on his associates' experiences with chlorophyll, he wrote, "It is interesting to note that there is not a single case recorded in which either improvement or cure has not taken place."[48] Later in 1941, *Reader's Digest* published an article called "The Green Magic of Chlorophyll," which discussed the tremendous potential of chlorophyll as a food and a medicine.[49]

"In the mid-1940's, however, the use of chlorophyll as medicine had reached its peak. Unfortunately, liquid chlorophyll turned out to be highly unstable; it could not be bottled and stored for more than a few hours. A synthetic chlorophyll extract, which was produced by fermenting fresh chlorophyll and bonding it with certain mineral elements proved to be inconsistent and at times caused negative side effects. Chlorophyll as a treatment was then abandoned by the medical profession, despite the dramatic effects indicated in various studies. Chlorophyll and many other natural antiseptics were replaced by faster-acting antibiotics and chemical antiseptics.

"Today, the importance of chlorophyll is receiving a great deal of renewed interest. One of chlorophyll's more important functions in the Hippocrates diet is oxygenation of the bloodstream. On a high-fat and high-protein diet, our oxygen supply is greatly reduced. Dr. John Gainer, reporting in the August 1971 issue of *Science News*, stated that even a moderate increase in blood-plasma protein can reduce oxygen levels of the blood by as much as 60 percent.[50] I have found that without sufficient oxygen in our blood, we develop symptoms of low energy, and sluggish digestion and metabolism. These outward signs are harbingers of serious illness to follow.

Deprived of an adequate supply of oxygen, the body becomes ripe for disease. In his book, *The Cause and Prevention of Cancer*, Dr. Otto Warburg, winner of a Nobel Prize for physiology and medicine, concluded that oxygen deprivation was a major cause of cancer and that with a steady supply of oxygen to all the cells, cancer could be prevented indefinitely.

B. Wheatgrass has Concentrated Chlorophyll

Wheatgrass, the grass grown from wheat berries (wheat seeds), is rich in chlorophyll, a substance nearly identical to the hemoglobin in human blood. Weight for weight wheatgrass has sixty times more vitamin C then oranges and eight times more iron then spinach. It has over a hundred vitamins, minerals and nutrients including a good source of vitamin B17. Wheatgrass contains concentrated chlorophyll, which is almost identical to the hemoglobin molecule in human blood. The only major difference between them is that the central atom in hemoglobin is iron; in chlorophyll, it is magnesium.

The Father of Wheatgrass is considered to be, Charles F. Schnabel (1895-1974) who researched and promoted it back in the 1940's, as noted by Steve Meyerowitz in his book on *Wheatgrass Nature's Finest Medicine*.[51]

In 1930's you could buy dried wheatgrass in pharmacies all across America, but that fell to the wayside as the pharmaceutical companies came into control. There is not enough money in it to pursue selling wheatgrass and the universities and pharmacies are looking for a way to make big money. But Ann Wigmore started growing it in the kitchen. The problem with straight wheatgrass juice is that you have to drink it right away because it degrades quickly thus most research is from dried products of wheatgrass. Barley grass is sister to wheat grass but barley is sweeter and less bitter in taste. Thus the flavor is better in barley then wheat grass. Another issue is that some people can't grow wheatgrass so powders are just as good.

"Ann Wigmore developed wheatgrass therapy and in most holistic clinic and health food stores it can be found. Wheatgrass juice along with raw foods, exercise, meditation and detoxification methods like juice fasting became the key elements in her program. "The body of the cancer patient must heal itself in the same way the physical body rebounds from a cut, bruise, or common cold," says Ann Wigmore, founder of the Hippocrates Health Institute in Boston. "The body must replace the lost cells with new cancer-free ones."[52]

Wheatgrass juice, it is claimed, helps to detoxify the body, eliminate dead tissue, and nourish the system. A nutritional program combining wheatgrass and 'live' foods (that is uncooked food - with enzymes and nutrients undamaged) is said to create optimal immune functioning, enabling the whole organism to reverse the cancer. Wheatgrass therapy has brought about striking recoveries from cancer. Yet many people in the alternative cancer field do not consider it a primary therapy." [53]

The scarcity of long term known survivors is explained by poor documentation and lack of follow-up. "We're into helping people, not into statistics - we're just not into documentation," a woman at the Health Institute in San Diego said. She said her Institute has many cases of long-term cancer survivors but that it does not give out names in order to respect clients' privacy.[54]

Dr. Ann Wigmore the discoverer of wheat grass and invented "nut milks" and dehydrated crackers, "almond loaf" and "live" candy. Dr. Ann discovered the many healing benefits of blending foods, a large part of which consisted of greens. She observed that eating blended food gave her superior health and cut her hours of sleep down to two hours per night.[55]

Along with wheatgrass therapy a 'live foods' diet was used to heal cancer. The term 'live food' was first applied by a Dr. Kristine Nolfi who healed herself of her malignant, fast growing breast cancer in the 1940's through a raw food diet. She later became the chief physician of the Humlegaarden sanatorium in Humlebaek, Denmark. There she treated patients with cancers of the breast, rectum, intestine, abdomen, stomach, lung and brain. "Patients suffering from cancer have generally suffered for many years from gastric catarrh and constipation. Cancer is the final stage in an over-acid and degenerated organism," wrote Dr. Nolfi. Her views are echoed today by the wheatgrass therapy movement in the United States.[56]

Gabriel Cousens, MD writes: "Primitive foods such as spirulina contain the highest food energy, the highest nutrient value, and use up the least amount of the planet's resources. Spirulina is also a powerful alkalinizing and healing food. It is an excellent support for the healing of hypoglycemia, diabetes, chronic fatigue, anemia, ulcers, and for boosting the immune system. It has been shown to repair free radical damage. Researchers have found it to contain a tumor necrosis factor. The anti-cancer power of spirulina is significant enough that at Harvard Medical School they found extracts of spirulina were extremely effective in treating cancer in hamsters."[57]

"A study by Annand (a) and another by Yarushalmy and Hilleboe (b), showed in various countries that the higher the level of vegetable consumption, the lower the level of heart disorders. Annand found that vegetable protein exerts a powerful protective action against arteriosclerosis in animal experiments."[58] "A low fat diet, maintained for a period of up to 3 years, failed to lower either the mortality or morbidity of patients suffering from arteriosclerosis (a) whereas after a period of only 4 to 5 weeks a diet high in fresh vegetables caused a significant reduction in this affliction. (b)"[59]

C. Healing with Chlorophyll

There are numerous healing benefits are written about of chlorophyll from cereal grass that can be considered. Here are a few of the many benefits and studies done on chlorophyll and related grasses.

Chlorophyll for treating cancer

Drs. F. Paloscia and G. Pollotten used chlorophyll therapy with some success in the **treatment of tuberculosis emphysema.**[60] **Cancer** [61] [62] [63] patients seem to have benefited to some degree from chlorophyll therapy, although results are inconclusive.

A Dr. Mahnaz Badamchian of the Dept. of Biochemistry and Molecular Biology, George Washing Univ., Medical Center found that **Anti-tumor properties** of barley leaf extract (BLE) on human prostrate, breast and melanoma cancer to significantly reduced. Badamchian states, this "could provide a novel nutritional approach to the treatment or prevention of cancer and present a potential breakthrough in cancer research."[64]

A study on wheat grass showed that it caused the inhibition of Carcinogens. "These results are of interest for two reasons: first, the **inhibition of activation of potent carcinogens** is quite strong at a reasonably low level of extract and second, the wheat sprout extract is nontoxic even at high levels while most known inhibitors are toxic at medium to high levels."[65]

Chlorophyll is non-toxic

Can there be such a beneficial tonic, completely safe, without side reactions? Toxicity studies [66] [67] [68] have shown that **chlorophyll is absolutely non-toxic** when administered parenterally (intravenous or intramuscular) or by mouth to animal and humans.   *Rev. Gastroentology; American Journal Surgery; Am. J. Med. Soc.*

Calcium is as good as milk

Greens such as kale, broccoli, and Bok choy are as good as milk in terms of calcium absorbability.[69]

Environmental Nutrition
The American Journal of Clinical Nutrition

Chlorophyll has no toxicity

"In hundreds of experiments and trials on humans and animals, chlorophyll therapy has always been shown to have **no toxic side effects**. Not just low toxicity. NO toxicity – whether ingested, injected or rubbed onto a surface. This fact alone makes chlorophyll one of the most unique therapeutic substances known to medical science."[70]

Chlorophyll heals wounds

"Chlorophyll heals wounds ... **stimulates repair of damaged tissues** and **inhibits growth of bacteria**. Medical literature is replete with reports demonstrating these effects. Surface wounds and sores due to surgery, compound fractures, osteomyelitis (bone inflammation), decubitus (bed sores), and routine cuts and scrapes all show fast and dramatic improvement with the topical use of chlorophyll. Chlorophyll therapy has saved limbs from amputation."[71] "D.H. Collings proved that chlorophyll therapy has a **shorter healing time of wounds**, shorter then with vitamin D, sulfanilamide, penicillin, or no treatment."[72]

Burns heal faster

"**Burns caused by heat, chemicals, and radiation heal faster** with chlorophyll therapy, whether or not they are infected, chlorophyll was used to prolong the survival of skin grafts before the development of immune-suppressing drugs which are now used."[73]

Peptic Ulcers heal faster

"Chlorophyll has also been shown to be **extremely effective in speeding the healing** of peptic ulcers, wounds which develop internally in the gastrointestinal tract. Several studies document the use of chlorophyll in the treatment of ulcers resistant to more conventional therapies. The results are quite impressive. In the Offenkrantz study, 20 of the 27 patients with chronic ulcers were relieved of pain and other symptoms in 24 to 27 hours. Complete healing of damaged tissues, as demonstrated by X-ray examination, occurred in 20 of 24 cases within two to seven weeks. These reports included case descriptions of dramatic recoveries from severe, long-standing problems."[74]

Promotes Regularity

"Chlorophyll tended to '**promote regularity**' in the patients studied. According to several investigators, chlorophyll did not act simply to stimulate bowel activity, as does a laxative. Rather, it promoted bowel regularity, stimulating bowel action only when the action was sluggish."[75]

Anti-inflammatory activities

"Japanese researchers have discovered a protein – P4-D1 – in barley grass juice that seems to protect cells from ultraviolet radiation and a specific carcinogen. This was said to be a result of the stimulation of DNA repair by this protein. Both the protein and another in barley grass juice – D1-G1 – have **been shown to have anti-inflammatory activity** when injected into lab animals. In addition, both these barley compounds are remarkably free from side effects."[76]

Prevents Liver from Making 'Bad' Cholesterol

Dr. Asaf Qureshi was a food consultant with the U.S. Department of Agriculture, did a study (1977) in which he "isolated an active compound in barley that suppressed the liver's ability to make cholesterol. This inhibitor is called tocotrienol – or Inhibitor 1, and two other inhibitors were found. These were found present in barley, rye and oats. All three inhibitors in barley deactivate an enzyme in the liver needed to make cholesterol. And they **suppressed the liver's ability to make LDL, the 'bad' cholesterol** which clogs the arteries, yet the 'good' cholesterol, HDL levels, remained intact. These three inhibitors in barley are also found in lesser amounts in other grains and vegetables. There is a cholesterol pill (Mevacor or lovastatin) that blocks an enzyme in the liver that stimulates the bad cholesterol (LDL) output."[77]

Relieves Chronic Constipation

In a study, "Israeli scientists tried substituting barley flour for wheat flour in biscuits and scones and gave them to 19 patients suffering from chronic constipation. Each patient was asked to eat three of the four barley biscuits a day. Fifteen of them **(79%) became completely free of constipation, had less gas and abdominal pain, and quit taking laxatives**. When they were deprived of these barley foods, virtually all the group became constipated and went back to laxatives within a month."[78]

Gluten Allergies

There is **no gluten in barley grass** and it can be used safely by people with gluten intolerance (celiac disease). Also the "chlorophyll in barley grass dilutes and enhances the elimination of gluten from the digestive system, according to one expert. According to John Heinerman, certain allergy specialists in southern California have been recommending green barley-juice powder, mixed with distilled water, to many of their gluten-sensitive patients."[79]

D. Chlorophyll a Brief History

Chlorophyll heals and cleanses all our organs and destroys man of our internal enemies, like pathogenic bacteria, fungus, cancer cells,[80] and others. "Chlorophyll has been proven helpful in preventing and healing many forms of cancer[81] and arteriosclerosis."[82] Chlorophyll has a long history and many advocates.

The following article by Jacob Handel, "Chlorophyll Supporter of all Human and Animal Life,"[83] (Hippocrates Institute magazine, "Healing Our World", FL, 2010), is an excellent historical overview of chlorophyll. There are many other journal studies and facts on chlorophyll, some related in this book which expand on this brief history.

It is known that "chlorophyll is a green pigment found in all plants, algae and cyanobacteria (blue-green algae). Vital for photosynthesis, chlorophyll allows plants to obtain energy from light by converting the sun's rays into chemical energy. Since all life on earth – with the exception of some bacteria – is supported by the sun, photosynthesis is a fundamental and essential process.

"In addition to its critical role in photosynthesis, chlorophyll is also a great indicator of the health attributes of foods. The deeper the green color of a plant food, the richer the food is in chlorophyll – and the more abundant the food is in health-building qualities. Foods rich in chlorophyll can play a role in blood production[84] and protection from cancer[85] [86] and radiation.[87] [88] Chlorophyll also has many therapeutic uses. Among these are wound healing,[89] intestinal regularity,[90] reducing cholesterol,[91] detoxification and deodorization. Chlorophyll is an especially unique way to address these issues because, through hundreds of experiments and trials on humans and test animals, chlorophyll therapy has always been shown to have no toxicity (absolutely zero toxic side effects) – whether ingested, injected or rubbed onto your skin.[92]

"Chlorophyll is built around a structure known as a porphyrin ring, which is common to a variety of natural organic molecules. Chief among these is hemoglobin, the substance in human and animal blood which carries oxygen from the lungs to the other tissues and cells of the body. When looking at the structures of heme (the oxygen carrying portion of hemoglobin), it's easy to see their similarities. The main difference between them is the porphyrin ring of hemoglobin is build around iron (Fe) and the porphyrin ring of chlorophyll is build around magnesium (Mg). Verdel first suggested the chemical similarity between hemoglobin and chlorophyll in 1855.[93]

"The similarity was specifically demonstrated in the early 1920's. Over the following twenty years, much research was done on inter-convertibility of the two substances in the body. While the process isn't quite as simple as substituting the magnesium molecule in chlorophyll with an iron molecule to turn it into hemoglobin, there is evidence of the blood-building characteristics of chlorophyll-rich foods. Studies supporting the correlation date as far back as the 1920's.

1926: Research suggested a **relationship between** the **chlorophyll** component pheophytin **and hemoglobin** generation.[94]

1933: Studies indicated that feeding chlorophyll-rich foods to rats triggered the **regeneration of red blood cells**.[95] Researchers demonstrated that this effect was not due to the iron or copper in the green foods.

1934: Dr. Rothemund discovered that porphyrins from chlorophyll **stimulated the synthesis of red blood cells** in a variety of animals when fed in small doses.[96]

1936: Drs. Hughes and Latner performed a study involving anemic rabbits. They fed the rabbits several doses and forms of chlorophyll. The doctors found that extremely small doses of purified chlorophyll or large doses of "a crude chlorophyll extract" produced "a very favorable effect on hemoglobin regeneration." The researchers went on to suggest, "the chlorophyll is acting as a physiological stimulant of the bone marrow and is not really concerned with the actual chemistry of regeneration of the porphyrin."[97] This study shows that chlorophyll found in food or very small purified amounts of **chlorophyll may stimulate the synthesis of red blood cells in the bone marrow**.

1936: Dr. Arthur Patek conducted a study in which fifteen patients with iron-deficiency anemia were fed different amounts of chlorophyll along with iron. Iron alone had already been shown to reverse this condition, but Patek demonstrated that when chlorophyll and iron were given together **the number of red blood cells and level of blood hemoglobin increased faster** than with iron alone. As stated by Dr. Patek, "This study may serve to encourage the use of a diet ample in greenstuffs and protein foods, for it must be that over a long space of time favorably nutritious elements are absorbed which aid the blood reserve and which furnish building stones for the heme pigments necessary to the formation of hemoglobin."[98] [99]

1970: Research indicates that some porphyrins (ringed structures in heme and chlorophyll) **stimulate the synthesis of globin (the protein portion of the hemoglobin molecule)**. This could partially explain the effect of chlorophyll on hemoglobin synthesis.[100]

"While the complex physiological processes involved in generating blood aren't completely understood, the parts of the process relating to nutrition are well defined. Essential nutrients for the maintenance of healthy blood include iron, copper, calcium, and vitamins C, B-12, K, A, folic acid, and pyridoxine, among others. **Many of these blood-building**

components are found in chlorophyll rich foods such as cereal glasses (wheat, oats, barley, etc.) and dark green vegetables.

"Young cereal plants absorb and synthesize vitamin K, vitamin C, folic acid, pyridoxine, iron, calcium and protein for their growth and development. These very same nutrients are essential to the generation and utilization of hemoglobin in humans and animals."[101]

Protection from Cancer
"Scientific evidence has shown that chlorophyll and the nutrients found in **green foods offer protection against toxic chemicals and radiation**. In 1980, Dr. Chiu Nan Lai at the University of Texas Medical Center reported that extracts of wheatgrass and other green vegetables inhibit the cancer-causing effects of two mutagens (benzopyrene and methylcholanthrene).[102] The more chlorophyll in the vegetable, the greater the protection from the carcinogen.

"Chlorophyll can reduce the ability of carcinogens to cause gene mutations, as shown in several laboratory studies. Chlorophyll-rich plant extracts, as well as water solutions of a chlorophyll derivative (chloropyllin), **dramatically inhibit the carcinogenic effects of common dietary and environmental chemicals**.[103] [104]

Protection from Radiation
"Green vegetables provide protection from radiation damage in test animals. This information has been reported in scientific literature dating back to the early 1950's. Early reports showed that certain vegetables significantly reduced mortality in rats exposed to lethal doses of X-rays.[105] Dark green broccoli offered more protection than the lighter green cabbage. In the later study, the same vegetables were shown to **reduce the damage caused by radiation**.[106] These protective effects were more pronounced when even darker green vegetables such as mustard greens and alfalfa leaves

were used. When two or more of the green vegetables were fed together, the positive resistance to radiation was greatest.

Chlorophyll vs. Chlorophyllin

"Chlorophyllin is a semi-synthetic sodium/copper derivative of chlorophyll. It has been used for over 50 years as a food additive and alternative medicine because it has a longer shelf life than natural chlorophyll and it cost less than some forms of natural chlorophyll. A 2005 study was conducted in the Netherlands to compare the effects of chlorophyll and chlorophyllin. Human diets high in red meats and low in green vegetables are associated with colon cancer. Such a diet was simulated in rats using dietary heme. The heme, simulating the red meat rich – and green vegetable lacking – diet of many people, caused a staggering increase in cytotoxicty (>50-fold increase, measured in fecal water), a nearly 100% increase in proliferation of colonocytes and almost complete inhibition of exfoliation of the colonocytes. The study found that chlorophyll, but not water-soluble chlorophyllins, completely prevented these heme-induced effects.

"While chlorophyllin has exhibited some of the same benefits as natural chlorophyll, this study shows that the natural option has an overwhelming advantage in at least one application. **The best way to incorporate more natural chlorophyll in your diet and reap all its wonderful health benefits is through green foods.** When you eat fresh, organic, chlorophyll-rich foods and drink their juices, you're getting the best of the best. Growing your own cereal grassed and juicing those costs pennies and these foods are the richest in chlorophyll."[107]

E. What are Green Food Supplements?

Green food supplements are one of the keys to health and healing nowadays it is a much easier and more efficient way to get greens into your diet in an optimum way. An article on the web by Mark Timon, C.S. (clinical nutrition)[108] the founder of Vibrant Health company which was one of the first to sell green powders, wrote about green foods and what they are about.

"I think it might be helpful to establish a definition of 'green foods' at the outset. Thirty plus years ago "green food" included only chlorophyll supplements. Later, wheat grass, barley grass, and their powders and juices expanded our understanding of green foods. Continuing up to today, a greater variety of nutritional raw materials derived from plants has become available as our industry has evolved. There are more new ones each year.

As a consequence, the definition of green foods can include, but is not necessarily limited to, all cereal grass (e.g. wheat, barley, oat, kamut, etc.) whole leaf powders, juice, and juice powders, green algae (e.g. chlorella), blue-green algae (e.g. spirulina), alfalfa, fresh water plants such as Hydrilla verticillata, and any other vegetable that is green. Okra, green beans, green peas, spinach, broccoli, kudzu, parsley, and zucchini are part of this list, as well as sprouts grown from their seeds.

Green food supplements, if properly formulated, can provide astonishing nutrient density. They can, in effect, return our dietary intake to something more closely approximating the richness of our ancestral, Paleolithic diet. (In the past everything was organic and industrial pollutants did not exist, way back in Paleolithic times thousands of years ago.) The import of this is significant, for few aspects of human biochemistry can function properly if trace nutrients are undersupplied, thereby making it harder to deal with the gluttonous portions of fat and carbohydrate present in modern diets.

The appeal lies in the simple fact that green foods are incredibly nutritious, with an actual power to heal. If each cell receives what it needs to function fully and efficiently, then the human body can, in many cases, re-establish normal biochemistry. Depending on the individual, the results might be a noticeable improvement in endurance, or faster recovery from exercise, to the eradication of a disease. Although green foods are usually not promoted as therapeutic supplements, the good ones will end up being so simply because they give the body what it needs to correct its own dysfunctions. The body heals itself, after all. Consumers are discovering these real benefits, and passing on the good news."

Chapter IV

Fiber and a Rainbow of Colors

A. The Rainbow of Smoothie Colors

Green smoothies are focused on the color green but there are numerous other colors in the rainbow. The majority of the scientific and experiential evidence is on the color green as this book has tried to show. There is a growing body of data about the health and healing effects of other colors. The primary reason for the color green is chlorophyll which has various products, mostly green powders from plants. There has been a great deal of health and healing benefits connected to chlorophyll.

Smoothies made of other colors rather than green are also encouraged but harder to prepare since adding darker colors like green or blue will overpower the lighter colors. Adding blueberries to a green smoothie will make it a darker green or bluish green color which is O.K. Thus we encourage making smoothies and eating a diet that has a rainbow effect of color.

There is a mosaic of colorful fruits and vegetables and the more colorful your food choices the better. Over the course of a week you want to maximize the colors on your plate. In the book, *The Color Code a Revolutionary Eating Plan for Optimum Health* by James Joseph, Ph.D.; Daniel Nadeau, M.D., Anne Underwood, they emphasize the importance of eating a variety of colors everyday for prevention and healing. The following material is basically from this work to show the importance of color.

"Indeed, almost every colorful food – from fresh-picked apples to cool green kiwis, bright red strawberries, and zesty, ripe oranges – is loaded with disease fighters. Many of them are found in the pigments themselves. Consider:

- The natural dye that makes tomatoes red may help ward off prostate cancer. A Harvard study found that 10 servings of tomato products a week reduced the risk of aggressive tumors by nearly half.
- The crimson in sour cherries may alleviate your arthritis pain. Researchers in Michigan found sour cherries to be 10 times stronger than aspirin.
- The yellow in corn could protect your eyesight. Repeated studies have found that it helps prevent macular degeneration, the leading cause of blindness in people over 65.
- The golden pigment in curry powder can reduce inflammation. Researchers are now studying its potential to prevent colon cancer, which is often linked to inflammation.
- The blue in bilberries, a close relative of blueberries, appears to enhance night vision.
- The indigo pigments in blueberries may starve off the natural mental decline that occurs as we age."[109]

Phytochemicals are not considered nutrients like proteins, fats, and carbohydrates and vitamins. Yet the term phytonutrient has started to be used along with phytochemical as scientists are become more aware of their great importance in the body. The majority of antioxidants and phytochemicals in our bodies have different uses for them then in plants. "The human body evolved with most of those chemicals," says botanist James Duke, author of *The Green Pharmacy* and compiler of a massive USDA phytochemical database. 'That's why you need them in your diet. Cancer in many cases is a deficiency of antioxidants. So is heart disease. Scientists are starting to think of these diseases as a shortage of phytochemicals."[110]

The pigments that give the color fall into two main classes known as Carotenoids and anthocyanins. These two are subgroups: the Carotenoids belong to a group of compounds called terpenes and terpenoids. Anthocyanins come from a group called Flavonoids which are part of a larger class known as polyphenolics.

The Carotenoids are the yellow-orange-red end of the spectrum. They are also found in leafy green vegetables but the strong color of green chlorophyll masks these other colors. In the fall in trees the cold pushes aside the chlorophyll and the golden hues of yellow, orange and red appear. "There are over 600 Carotenoids in nature, but only 50 in the human diet – of which 25 or so get into the bloodstream. The most important of these are alpha- and beta-carortene, beta-cryptoxanthin, lycopene, lutein, and zeaxanthin."[111]

The other major class of pigments found throughout the plant kingdom, are the anthocyanins which have hues ranging from crimson and magenta to violet and indigo. "Anthocyanins are also widely distributed in the food we eat. Cherries, plums, red currants, and blueberries all owe their beautiful hues to anthocyanins. There are more than 300 of these pigments, 70 of which have been reported in fruits."[112]

Scientists are still learning what all the phytochemicals are all about and how they work in their vast synergistic networks. Even though they can be dehydrated some of the beneficial benefits can be lost. The best way to get all these benefits is by eating living foods in various color combinations. "'There are thousands of compounds in plants that are associated with lower disease rates,' says Cornell University biochemist T. Colin Campbell, who helped conduct the longest running study to date of the Chinese die and disease prevention. The only way to take advantage of them all is by eating a diet rich in brightly colored fruits and vegetables, not popping supplements every day. Says Campbell: 'There are no magic bullets.'"[113]

The more colorful the vegetable often means the more nutrients and the better for you. "Virtually all fruits and vegetables – pale and vibrant alike – have something to recommend them. But vegetables that are darker not only have more antioxidant pigments – they often have more vitamins as well. For example:

- Butternut squash delivers more carotenes – and hence, more vitamin A – than summer squash, which is essentially white on the inside.
- Pink grapefruit give you the antioxidants lycopene and beta-carotene, which are missing from white grapefruit.
- Deep green romaine lettuce contains more B vitamins than pale iceberg. 'Eat a whole cup of iceberg and you get ten percent of the U.S. Recommended Daily Allowance for ... well, nothing," says nutritionist Bonnie Liebman of the Center for Science in the Public Interest.
- Even red wine packs a more potent antioxidant punch than white."[114]

To optimize your nutrition shopping for color is best; maximize colors of the produce you buy. "Any fruit or vegetable you buy should be the one with the best color – the reddest strawberries, the blackest blackberries. Shop for broccoli that is a deep, dark green, not tinged with yellow." There are two reasons for shopping for the best colors.

"First, as fruits ripen, the pigments themselves become denser. Blueberries double and triple their anthocyanin content between the time they first turn blue and the time they reach full maturity. Sour cherries show a twentyfold increase. Second, as fruits and vegetables ripen, they increase their stores of vitamins and minerals. By buying the bright crimson strawberries rather than pale, half green ones, you'll not only get more anthocyanins, you'll get more vitamin C, too."[115]

Even though there's not a lot of evidence of eating a colorful diet is a healing diet, it can be said: "There is, however, one statement that we can make with absolute certainty. A low-fat diet that includes a healthy dose of fruits and vegetables can save lives. That's been shown time and time again.

- A powerful Harvard study found that out of 114,000 doctors and nurses, those who consumed five to six servings of produce a day reduced their risk of stroke by 31 percent, compared with those who ate the least of these foods.
- A study of 800 older Dutch men found that those who consumed the most onions, apples and tea lowered their risk of fatal heart attacks by 70 percent over those who consumed the least.
- Based on numerous studies, the American Institute for Cancer Research estimates that a diet rich in fruits and vegetables could reduce cancers by 30 to 40 percent.
- 'What's crystal clear is that populations who exercise regularly and eat low-fat, high-produce diets have multiple health benefits,' says Dr. Michael Thun, vice president of the American Cancer Society. 'These include reduced risks of heart attack and stroke, diabetes, obesity, and various cancers. It's that simple.'"[116]

Phytochemicals and antioxidants are a major reason why fruits and vegetables deserve so much attention. Dr. Joseph and Dr. Nadeau write: "By including antioxidants in your diet, you can help reduce 'oxidative stress,' or the damage caused by oxygen radicals. Ronald Prior, who helped devise the ORAC test, recommends consuming at least 3,500 ORAC units a day. That's not hard if you start with a serving or two of strawberries. Here is a list of the top antioxidant foods that Prior and Cuohua Cao have tested so far. The ORAC values of individual fruits and vegetables can vary, according to growing conditions.

Dried Fruits	ORAC	Seasonings	ORAC
Prunes	5,770	Garlic	1,939
Raisins	2,830		
Fresh Fruits		Vegetables and Legumes	
Blueberries	2,400	Watercress	2,223
Blackberries	2,036	Kale	1,770
Cranberries	1,750	Spinach, raw	1,260
Strawberries	1,540	Asparagus	1,241
Raspberries	1,220	Brussels sprouts	980
Plums	949	Alfalfa sprouts	930
Avocado	782	Broccoli florets	890
Oranges	750	Beets	840
Red grapes	739	Red bell peppers	731
Cherries	670	Kidney beans	460

Dried fruits and garlic are listed separately because they contain relatively little water and therefore have an unfair advantage when ORACs are considered on an ounce-for-ounce basis. These are measured in ORAC units per 100 grams (about 3.5 ounces) of food. Sources: Boxin Ou, Brunswick Labs (watercress and asparagus); Ronald Prior and Guohua Cao, USDA-Agricultural Research Service (all other foods).

     The best way to eat all these foods is just as nature made them, in the least processed form available. Thus whole apples are better than apple juice. Whole strawberries are better than strawberry jam. Baked potatoes are better than potato chips which have been peeled, chopped, fried and salted. This is because the healthy outer skins are stripped away; sugar and salt are added; some are cooked and processed with various chemicals and preservatives. Try to eat a kaleidoscope of colors in the life-giving vegetables. Thus when you get a salad get a whole plate of various colors to maximize the nutrient and phytonutrient value of the meal.

B. Fiber in Smoothies

Victoria Boutenko in *Green for Life* has some good comments on fiber. Dr. Bernard Jensen, D.C., Ph.D. a nutrition expert stated: "Any cleansing program such begin in the colon ... In the 50 years I've spent helping people to overcome illness, disability and disease, it has become crystal clear that poor bowel management lies at the root of most people's health problems. In treating over 300,000 patients, it is the bowel that invariably has to be cared for first before any effective healing can take place."[117]

Fiber is a major influence in elimination and there are two main types of fiber: soluble and insoluble. Both are abundantly found in fruits and vegetables. Fiber is like a broom and sweeps out the intestines and colon among other things. Increasing fiber has a long list of medical improvements.

A famous French doctor of Natural Hygiene, Albert Mosseri, has conducted over 4,000 long-term water fasts at his clinic. "He came to the extraordinary conclusion that long-term fast were a 'risky waste of time.' He now oversees much shorter water fasts followed by what he calls 'half-fasts,' in which he introduces a limited amount of food rich in fiber in addition to water. During this important stage of healing, his patients receive only one pound of fruits and one pound of vegetables daily until their elimination is complete.[118] Dr. Mosseri states that switching to this 'half-fast' method has accelerated elimination to such a degree that 100% of his patients develop profound signs of a deep cleansing process in the form of a dark coating of their tongue, often charcoal black or dark brown."[119]

Victoria Boutenko states that: "The U.S. recommended daily allowance for fiber is 30 grains per day. The average American consumes between 10 and 15 grams of fiber a day.[120] That is far from sufficient. . . . I believe we should consume 50 to 70 grams of fiber per day or more. However, we have to increase the intake of fiber gradually. It can be dangerous to switch overnight from 10 grams to 70.

Many of our bodies have degenerated over the decades due to the consumption of processed foods. In addition, we have adopted many unnatural practices like lack of exercise and spending most of the time indoors. Therefore, we need to reintroduce healthy habits into our life slowly to give our body time to readjust. Green smoothies are perfect for this gradual shift."[121]

The body's ability to heal itself and maintain normal health is greatly dependent upon the homeostasis of the body. Homeostasis is the physiological process that keeps all substances in the body at the levels necessary for optimal health. The homeostasis of the body depends greatly on the endocrine system, which releases hormones to almost every cells, organ and function in the body.

"To make it really simple, the endocrine system in a human body acts like a factory combined with a supermarket that manufactures and supplies every substance requested by any gland or organ at any time, in any needed quantity. What would such factory need? An abundance of high quality supplies! Similarly, the endocrine system in our body absolutely needs all nutrients, including vitamins, amino acids, carbohydrates, essential fatty acids, minerals and all trace elements. Supplying all of these nutrients to our body is critical for good health.

Greens match all these purposes better than any other food! Once again, when blended, the nutrients from greens are absorbed more efficiently and provide many times more nutrients than other foods and even traditionally made salads. In other words, by drinking green smoothies we support our homeostatic balance in the most optimal way."[122]

Victoria gives a good example of the difference between the complex proteins found in animals' products to the individual amino acids, found in fruits, vegetables and in greens. In addition keep in mind that meat-based amino acids have a double helix bond that holds them together, whereas plant-based amino acids have a single helix bond in the molecular structure.

"It is clear that the body has to work a lot less when creating protein from the assortment of individual amino acids from greens, rather than the already combined, long molecules of protein , assembled according to the foreign pattern of a totally different creature such as a cow or a chicken. I would like to explain the difference between complex proteins and individual amino acids with a simple anecdote.

"Imagine that you have to make a wedding dress for your daughter. Consuming the complex proteins that we get from cows or other creatures is like going to the second hand store, and buying many other people's used dresses, coming home and spending several hours ripping apart pieces of the dresses that you like and combining them into a new dress for your daughter. This alternative will take a lot of time energy and will leave a great deal of garbage. You could never make a perfect dress this way.

"Consuming individual amino acids is like taking your daughter to a fabric store to buy beautiful new fabric, lace, button, ribbons, threads, and pearls. With these essential elements you can make a beautiful dress that fits her unique body perfectly. Similarly, when you eat greens, you 'purchase' new amino acids, freshly made by sunshine and chlorophyll, which the body will use to rebuild its parts according to your own unique DNA.

"Contrary to this, your body would have a hard time trying to make a perfect molecule of protein out of something else's molecules, which consist of totally different

48

combinations of amino acids. Plus, your body would most likely receive a lot of unnecessary pieces that are hard to digest. These pieces would be floating around in your blood like garbage for a long time, causing allergies and other health problems. Professor W.A. Walker from the Department of Nutrition at the Harvard School of Public Health, states that, 'Incompletely digested protein fragments may be absorbed into the blood stream. The absorption of these large molecules contributes to the development of food allergies and immunological disorders."[123]

Professor T. Colin Campbell of Cornell University notes: "There is a mountain of compelling evidence showing that so called 'low-quality' plant protein, which allows for slow but steady synthesis of new proteins, is the healthiest pure type of protein."[124] After a chapter of explaining the abundance of proteins in greens, Victoria Boutenko concludes: "In summary, greens provide protein in the form of individual amino acids. These amino acids are easier for the body to utilize than complex proteins. A variety of greens can supply all the protein we need to sustain each of our unique bodies."[125]

C. Grains vs. Sprouted Grains

Grains grown in a farm setting have only been around for the last 10,000 years, since the agricultural revolution. Our original gene structure is not designed for grain products, that's why different grains give us so many health problems. A vegan diet cuts out animal products and a raw vegan diet cuts out all or most grain products, if not sprouted. Grains in the past were used as animal foods. The raw food movement uses minimal grains or no grains at all, unless they are sprouted. This is a difference between being a vegan and a raw vegan.

Most raw food writers and chefs, in the 1990 to 2005 publications emphasized no grains for the raw vegan diet including:

Gabriel Cousens,[126] Doug Graham,[127] David Wolfe,[128] Victoria Boutenko,[129] Rhio,[130] Chad Sarno,[131] Juliano,[132] Nomi Shannon,[133] Elizabeth Baker,[134] Frederic Patenaude,[135] Brenda Cobb,[136] Charlie Trotter and Roxanne Klein,[137] Shazzie,[138] Alex Ferrara,[139] Elaine Love,[140] Igor Boutenko,[141] Sergei and Valya Boutenko,[142] Julie Wandling.[143] Paul Nison,[144] Stephen Arlin,[145] Robert Young,[146] Brian Clement,[147] Anna Maria Clement,[148] Cherie Soria,[149] James Tibbetts,[150] Brigitte Mars,[151] James Levin, Natalie Cederquist,[152] Jeremy Safron & Renee Underkoffler,[153] Rita Romano,[154] Annie Padden Jubb and David Jubb,[155] Jeremy Safron,[156] Elysa Markowitz,[157] Johann Schnitzer[158] Charlotte Gerson[159] Jameth Dina,[160] George Malkmus,[161] Ronda Malkmus.[162] Alissa Cohen, Roe Gallo, Harvey Diamond, Marilyn Diamond.[163] Melissa Diane Smith (a nutritionist has a whole book on the ill effects of grains in a diet).[164] "

Some believe that too much food from grains (starches, cereals) burden the digestion, cause acidosis and impure blood, arthritis, cancer, other metabolic problems and are considered to be the chief factors in skin disorders. One health author, Ross Horne, cites, "Some doctors, who had spent their entire careers in the study of degenerative diseases, were specifically opposed to the use of cereals as suitable foods in the human diet."[165]

Sprouting brings grains alive, they become living foods and not dormant or dead foods. Let me cite a few experts on this topic. Brenda Cobb notes: 'Let's talk about the difference in raw and Living Foods. Raw foods are those picked off trees or vines, such as apples, berries, cucumbers, avocados, squash, tomatoes and bananas, etc. Living Foods are beans, grains, nuts, and seeds that have been soaked and sprouted. When the sprout comes out of the grain, seed or berry, it becomes a "Living Food," full of life and increased nutritional value. Ann Wigmore made the point about this being the Living Foods Lifestyle.'"[166]

Gabriel Cousens, MD, a leading raw food expert, gives a good insight into the scientific basis for soaking and sprouting: "In the Conscious Eating Kitchen (his facilities kitchen), all of the nuts, seeds and grains we use are sprouted and/or soaked. Soaking and sprouting serve several important functions. First, nutrients begin to be broken down into their simplified form. For example, proteins begin the process of breaking down into amino acids, carbohydrates into simple sugars, fats into fatty acids, while minerals chelate or combine with proteins. This significantly improves digestion and assimilation, and it is why soaked or sprouted foods are considered predigested."[167]

Dr. Cousens continues: "Second, the actual content of nutrients dramatically increases during soaking and sprouting process. Proteins, vitamins, enzymes, and minerals increase 300 to 1200%. For example, zinc present in alfalfa sprouts increases from approximately 6.8 mg per 100 grams of seed to 18 mg per 100 grams dried weight in the sprout. One cup of alfalfa sprouts provides twice the US RDA for zinc. Enzyme inhibitors, phytic and oxalic acids, and mineral chelates are washed away during the soaking and sprouting process. These chemicals function as natural defenses against bacterial, fungal, insect and animal predators in the growing process of the plant, but many interfere with digestion and assimilation when consumed. Finally, chlorophyll develops in the sprouts as they turn green."[168]

It's a lot more than just increased nutritional value. Dr. Gabriel Cousens notes: "Grains constitute the next class of yeast/fungi/mold-stimulating foods after the high-sugar foods and fruits in particular. Research shows that stored grains ferment in ninety days. Within that time many mycotoxins are produced. In essence, stored grains are a mycotoxic hazard. A correlation was found between 112 patients with esophageal cancer and eating of stored grains (*Cancer, 1987*). There was a particular risk factor for stomach cancer among Scandinavian and German men eating stored grains reported in *The Fungal/Mycotoxin Etiology of Human Disease*, vol. 2. Stored potatoes also represent a mycotoxic risk. The black spots on them are caused by the fungi aspergillums and fusarium, which produce the mycotoxins aflatoxin and fumosium. Some grains are not stored and therefore are not a mycotoxin hazard. These include pelt, amaranth, quinoa, millet, buckwheat, and wild rice. Buckwheat is often thought of as a seed, but it is actually classified as a grain."[169]

In the book, *Going Against the Grain*, it notes: "Many nutritionists recommend whole grains in place of refined grains, and at first thought, this sounds like good dietary advice. On paper at least, whole grains contain more nutrients. They also have more blood sugar-regulating fiber. Because of that fiber, they generally rank lower on the glycemic index and offer more protection against Type 2 diabetes and heart disease than refined grains.[170] [171] (citing[2]) However, whole grains have numerous nutritional shortcomings that make these foods far less beneficial to health than they've been made out to be. Their key nutritional downfalls include high carbohydrate content, anti-nutrients that impair the absorption of minerals such as calcium, iron, and zinc, and lectins that wreak havoc with intestinal and immune function. The more that whole grains are eaten, the more their nutritional shortcomings aggravate body function and lead to serious head problems. Ironically, many people switch from a high-refined grain diet to a high whole-grain diet in a search for better health but actually set themselves up for conditions such as bone problems, iron-deficiency anemia, and autoimmune conditions.'"[172]

---

[2] *(Journal of the American Medical Association; American Journal of Clinical Nutrition)*

Dr. Vivian Virginia Vetrano, a raw fooder since the early 70's, sums up the problems with grains: 'We all know that people can live on them, but the question is, can people actually be superbly healthy by partaking of grains, especially a lot of them? The answer is no. A diet of pure grains is acid-forming, and it does not supply the proper proportion of the alkaline minerals to balance the acidic ones.'"[173]

Learning to sprout regular seeds like alfalfa seeds is an easy way to learn how to sprout. Sprouting is considered a superfood and is a part of a raw vegan or Living Foods lifestyle. One raw fooder, Steve Meyerowitz is known as the Sproutman and has written a book on *Sprouts the Miracle Food*,[174] and he sells a sprouting machine that sprouts seeds and other foods automatically. There are others that have different approaches but it is all about bringing the dormant grain products and other foods Alive!

D. Cooking Destroys Nutrients

One of the reasons the green smoothie revolution took off was because of the chlorophyll making up the greens, but another major reasons is that smoothies are not cooked; they are primarily if not totally raw foods. Cooking can destroy or denature the chlorophyll in the foods.

Heating to above 120 degrees destroys all the enzymes. Heating above 150 degrees destroys all the water soluble vitamins (such as the B complex). Heating to boiling at 212 degrees is what starts to denature the protein and other nutrients. For instance if you fry or boil two eggs about 50% of the protein is lost, so you only have the protein that is equivalent to one egg.

Some interesting facts/thoughts to ponder on for cooking are the following:

Cooking, baking roasting, broiling, boiling and steaming destroy from 30% to 90% of the nutrition in the food, resulting in a nutrient-deficient diet, the main cause of degenerative diseases. 100% of the enzymes are destroyed in cooking. Minerals are lost when cooking; liquids (broth) are poured out.

Cooked foods become so devitalized they take more energy than they give and are difficult to digest.

Cooked foods shorten our life span.

Cooked foods cause far more build-up of toxins, a factor suppressing the immune system and making the body more susceptible to disease of all kinds.

Cooked foods encourage over eating, resulting in weight gain. Since they are nutrient-deficient, they leave the system still hungering for and craving food.

The natural fiber is broken down, increasing transit time of food through the gastrointestinal tract. Increased transit time means sugars ferment, proteins putrefy, and fats turn rancid, loosening toxins for absorption.

The carcinogenic charcoal forms during some cooking procedures.

Leucocytosis (an increase in white blood cell count and associated with a pathological condition) increases upon ingestion of cooked food.

There is poor mastication resulting in decreased saliva and enzyme flow; food is, therefore, poorly prepared for digestion.

Cooked food is most often fragmented/refined/deficient.

Cooked food is most often highly chemicalized.

Cooked food is prepared in utensils that give off toxic metal/plastic/paint particles.

Cooked food is most often addicting and promotes overeating.

Finally cooked foods falsely satisfy the taste and appetite but cause abnormal cravings for sugary foods (candy, cakes, pies, ice creams, cookies, etc.) Heavy meats, richly-seasoned starches, such as breads with spreads, deep fat-fried potato and corn chips, French fries, spicy, rich grain and legume dishes also cause abnormal cravings. After such a meal, the coffee drinker craves coffee, which over-stimulates the pancreas to produce more enzymes to digest all the heavy food.[175]

Supermarkets are places where many foods are dead foods that lie in state, laid out for the public to see and choose. Outside of the produce department, almost everything in a supermarket is dead or dormant food stuffs. People need to shift from dead foods towards living foods, not the dead, dormant and dying foods they've been eating for years. In the produce department, all the fruits and vegetables are Living Foods, and in the frozen foods section there are some living/frozen foods.

Chapter V

The Alkaline Body and Oxygen

A. Alkaline Forming Foods

Every doctor across the country should be telling their patients to be eating an "alkaline forming" diet! And a vegetarian diet is one of the best alkaline forming diets!

Distilled water is 7.0 pH and human milk is 7.43 pH which is the basis for man's normal pH. Thus our diet needs to be on the alkaline side of things to stay healthy. But the Standard American Diet is highly acidic and works off the 'extremes' found mostly in animal food and plant derivatives. Cooking is a form of food processing and is generally more acid forming. Raw foods are more alkalizing and cleansing for the body particularly after an extreme diet like the unhealthy Standard American Diet. The homeostasis of the body seeks a 7.4 pH and other constant conditions such as a body temperature of 98.6 degrees F, certain glucose levels in the blood, certain amounts of body fluids etc.

Theodore A. Baroody, N.D., D.C., Ph.D. points out, that: "Unfortunately, waste acids that are not eliminated when they should be are reabsorbed from the colon into the liver and put back into general circulation. They then deposit in the tissues. It is these tissue residues that determine sickness or health! Discover what tissue acid wastes are present and begin the process of alkalizing yourself, thus ridding them from the body. The result will be superior health, energy and strength to enjoy life fully. He further points out, "To replenish and sustain your alkaline reserves, follow the Rule of 80/20 – which means to eat 80% of your foods from the alkaline-forming list and 20% from the acid-forming list. Research, clinical experience, and the knowledge of the 'greats' in nutrition, have re-confirmed this ideal ratio of 80/20%."[176]   In a footnote, he indicates that 99.85% of the people should have this ratio but people in extremely hot places like the Sahara desert may need a more alkaline-forming diet and people in the North or South Pole may require a more acid forming diet in the long winters.

Dr. Robert Young PhD. in his book, *Sick and Tired Reclaim Your Inner Terrain*, explains pH in the role of health and healing. "Most people today understand environmental pollution and how it sickens the Earth: we live off the planet and pollute it with waste. Well, illness is basically the same thing. These morbidly evolved organisms are literally eating us alive and polluting us. The thing is, we pollute ourselves first, thus creating the one physiological disease: pH imbalance/toxicity in our terrain. Toxins and an acid-forming diet disrupt body chemistry, and this loss of balance (i.e., dis-ease) in turn disturbs the central balance of the microzyma. Nutritional deficiencies can have the same effect, but can also be created by acidification: the evolution of microzymas is into bacteria and ultimately into a yeast and fungus Y/F infestation. Y/F can infest the blood and any cell or tissue, causing different symptoms.

"As more acid wastes back up and the body slowly stews in its own poisonous wastes, the acid begins to corrode veins, arteries, cells and tissues, leading to high valence cellular disorganization, which the medical community refers to as degenerative disease."[177] "Normal body function and health require adequate alkaline reserves as well as the correct pH in tissues and blood. A major means of ensuring these conditions is the proper dietary ratio of alkaline to acid foods. A ratio of at least 80% to 20% - four parts alkaline to one part acid - is required (possibly 3 to 1 for a healthy person). When the proper ratio is maintained, morbid microforms are discouraged."[178]

A mistake that is common is people assume that they should eat only alkaline foods and not acidic but it is what happens to the food inside the body that counts. Thus a person needs to look at whether the foods are "acid forming" or "alkaline forming" in the body. A good example are acidic fruits such as limes and lemons which are very acidic outside the body but inside the body they promote alkalinity. One of the reasons for this is that they contain minerals such as calcium, potassium and magnesium which are very alkalizing to the body.

There are different ways that the body can maintain pH levels; the major route is through minerals from the diet. Alkalizing minerals include: calcium, magnesium, potassium and iron. The blood has to maintain a constant 7.4 pH or the person could go unconscious or die. Thus the blood is buffered to stay between 7.35 to 7.45 pH. One of the reasons for this is maintaining enough oxygen in the blood to circulate it to the rest of the body; another reason is that the heart could cease to beat if it did not stay in that range.[179] Cancer of the heart is unknown because of the constant level of oxygen in the blood and the constant alkaline pH.

In order to maintain this constant pH the body will sacrifice other parts of the body mostly the bones. This is a primary cause for osteoporosis and is shown in many studies (see section D - Strict Vegetarian, 59-63). The whole body suffers in an acidic condition and numerous degenerative diseases thrive in this environment. This is one of the primary reasons why vegetarian diets have been so successful involved in the process of healing cancer.

The lactic acid found in acidic bodies and given off when a person has cancer can damage the DNA and RNA which are the control mechanism of growth. Once these mechanisms are damaged the cells can multiply out-of-control. Thus not only do they damage the DNA but contribute to a low-oxygen environment.

Changing to a vegetarian diet can over time change the pH but when a person has cancer they need to be on a

58

strict vegetarian diet, preferably a raw vegan diet and at least initially use some supplements, mineral supplementation, to help change the pH over faster. Raw fruits and vegetables have an abundance of alkalizing minerals and they are alkaline-forming in the body which is the important thing.

Degenerative diseases grow in an acidic environment. Cancer is a prime example. Cancer cells thrive in bodies that are acidic. And after the body has cancer it becomes even more acidic because of the cancer because lactic acid is a by-product of cancer cell metabolism that causes the cellular environment to become more acidic then before. Cancer does not like oxygen and overly acidic bodies have less oxygen the alkaline tissues. The anaerobic nature of cancer cells is why cancer grows best in acidic tissues. Dr. Sherry Rogers, when she discusses how cancer cells become like yeast cells with a low pH (very acidic); "The normal pH of a cancer cell is 6.5, while a normal cell is 7.4. As soon as the pH of a cancer cell reaches 7.0, it stops growing; a little higher and it starts dying."[180] "According to *Cell Society*, by Dr. S. Okada, cancer cells grow well in a culture solution produced by the metabolic wastes of regular cells. Since the metabolic waste material of regular cells is acidic, cancer cells, then, like this acidic condition."[181]

The enzymes in the body are some of the best defenses. Such as the pancreatic enzymes seek out and destroy tumors and other foreign matter. These enzymes are weaken and do not work as well in an acidic environment. Meat and dairy are very acidic adding to this problem, and the pancreatic enzymes are used up trying to breakdown the meat (a foreign substance and not seen as real food) instead of going to attack the cancer cells. This shows the need for a strict vegetarian diet during cancer therapy. Animal products such as meat, fish, poultry and eggs are very acid-forming in the body and give off by-products such as phosphoric acid, sulphuric acid, and uric acid.

Fast growing and slow growing tumors have been correlated to its usage of anaerobic functioning, which is directly related to pH. The National Cancer Institute found in experiments that: "the more aggressive (fast-growing) a cancer was, the higher its glucose fermentation rate was, and the slower-growing a cancer was, the lower its fermentation rate was."[182] In other words the more acidic the body the faster the cancer will grow, especially the more aggressive cancers.

Even though mineral supplementation can help do this a physicist Aubrey Brewer, Ph.D. (1893-1986) came up with an approach to use "cesium" which is the most alkaline (or alkalizing) of all the elements. He published his findings in *Pharmacology Biochemistry and Behavior*.[183] This raises the intercellular pH which kills the cancer cells. This method works faster than the use of diet and supplementation. Cancer cells thrive in highly acidic extracellular fluids and do not grow best in alkaline fluids. Whereas Dr. Brewers approach works mostly on the intracellular fluids, a strict vegetarian diet should be used along with it to support the therapy in the extracellular fluids of the cancer cells and around the body in general.[184] By changing the pH of the cancer cell towards "weak alkalinity" (a pH of 8 or so), "the survival of the cancer cell is endangered." In addition, acidic and toxic materials, normally formed in the cancer cells, could be "neutralized and eliminated."[185]

Back in 1931 Otto Warburg was awarded the Nobel Prize for his discovery that cancer is caused by weakened cell respiration due to a lack of oxygen at the cellular level. "According to Warburg, damaged cell respiration causes fermentation, resulting in low pH (acidity) at the cellular level. Dr. Warburg, in his Nobel Prize winning study, illustrated the environment of the cancer cell. A normal healthy cell undergoes an adverse change when it can no longer take in oxygen to convert glucose into energy. In the absence of oxygen, the cell reverts to a primal nutritional program to nourish itself by converting glucose through the process of fermentation. The lactic acid produced by fermentation lowers the cell pH (acid/alkaline balance) and destroys the ability of DNA and RNA to control cell division. The cancer cells then begin to multiply. The lactic acid simultaneously causes severe local pain as it destroys cell enzymes. Cancer appears as a rapidly growing external cell covering, with a core of dead cells.

Otto Warburg won the Nobel Prize for showing that cancer thrives in anaerobic (without oxygen), or acidic, conditions. In other words, the main cause for cancer is acidity of the human body. Dr. Otto Warburg finished one of his most famous speeches with the following statement: '... nobody today can say that one does not know what cancer and its prime cause is. On the contrary, there is no disease whose prime cause is better known, so that today ignorance is no longer an excuse that one cannot do more about prevention.'"[186]

Victoria Boutenko notes that, "Fats as the main contributor to weight gain is a popular delusion among dieters. This misconception leads to massive confusion and explains why so many overweight people are not succeeding in losing weight. I am sure that many people would be shocked to find out that we may gain weight from eating, say, cheese, not only because it is rich in fat, but mostly due to its high acidic level. In response to high pH acid, the body creates fat cells to store the acid. For example, almonds have 70% fat, and pork has only 58%. However, pork has one of the highest acid values, -38, while almonds are alkaline forming, +3. This is why it is so crucial to know, in addition to nutritional value, the pH index. Knowing the pH indexes of various foods can help us balance our personal daily meal plans."[187]

The so-called "bad" cholesterol, lipoprotein (LDL) is made by the liver in order to bind the toxins and deactivate the acidic waste that comes from certain foods, such as fats and animal protein.[188]

Victoria Boutenko points out her own experience where she tried using litmus paper to measure her pH levels and encouraged her family to do so too. "However, every time I measured my saliva or urine, it was almost always acid. ... Since I started drinking green smoothies, I decided to check my pH balance once again. I tested both my salvia and urine and was surprised to see that my litmus paper was now the stable green color of alkalinity!" It was then that Victoria clearly understood the "tight connection between the food that we intake and our pH balance." "After staying so many years on a 100% raw diet, I have come to the conclusion that it is impossible to maintain a good alkaline pH balance without consuming large quantities of dark leafy greens, approximately two bunches or one to two pounds every day."[189]

The human body adapts and changes its biochemistry and taste buds as our diet changes. Victoria notes how she had a hard time drinking wheatgrass juice when she was raw but after she started drinking green smoothies for a year she was able to drink wheatgrass and loved it. Wheatgrass juice consists of 70% chlorophyll and contains about 92 different minerals, beneficial enzymes, vitamins (B, C, E, H and K) and 19 amino acids. Barley grass, alfalfa and other cereal grasses also have a lot of benefits like the benefits of wheatgrass. The high oxygen content and mineral content in chlorophyll helps to make it very alkalizing as a food source.

There is a psychological factor involved in pH levels. Some factors that make people more acidic are stress, loud noises or music, speaking or hearing harsh words, bitter words, being angry and upset, over working or over-exercising, worrying, some T.V. shows or other nerve racketing experiences and many others.

Then there are psychological factors that make people more alkaline such as laughter and jokes, smiles, hugs, hearing compliments, classical or quiet music, watching and listening to fun, healthy audio or visual entertainment, being in nature, singing, praying, meditating, friendly conversations and many others.

B. Growing Fresh Air - Oxygen

A way to get more oxygen naturally is through a greenhouse. Have you ever walked through an enclosed greenhouse and taken a deep breath to experience the oxygen in the air? A lot of plants give off a lot of oxygen which is noticeable whether in a greenhouse or your bedroom. If you put a lot of big leafy plants in your bedroom or living room they would give off a lot of oxygen and also clean the air in the room. This higher level of oxygen in the air would increase the oxygen you breathe into your body. This would help to build your immune system and fight the cancer.

Another way to get more oxygen into the body is through drinking a lot of freshly made juices. At the Gerson clinic they emphasis 13 glasses of freshly made raw juice every day, one glass every hour. Of course there are several reasons for this with all the nutrients and phytonutrients that are being put into the body through the juice. But one reason that is often overlooked is the amount of extra oxygen that is taken in. When juice is freshly made a lot of oxygen ends up being attached to the molecules in the juice which is transported to the cells in the body.   These added oxygen molecules in the cellular structure of the freshly made juice are given off in the body raising the level of oxygen in the body naturally. This extra oxygen is a major problem for cancer cells and helps to defeat the cancer cells.

Whether 13 glasses a day are needed or 6 glasses a day would be enough is up for debate. But the important thing is that the juice is freshly made. The longer fresh juice is keep the more it oxidizes and loses its oxygen! Ideally you should drink the juice right after it is made.

Another well known way to get oxygen into the body is to exercise. There are many types of exercise that can do this, one good one is yoga. Yoga involves a lot of stretching of the muscles and deep breathing which brings oxygen into those muscles, glands and areas of the body worked on. But perhaps long walks could also be helpful. A cancer patient needs to take the time to exercise and breathe deeply.

Growing fresh air happens when you have plants in your house or work place. The U.S. Environmental Protection Agency (EPA) currently ranks (1996) indoor air pollution as one of the top five threats to public health. Low relative-humidity levels are also associated with poor IAQ. Healthy humidity levels range between 35 and 65 percent. Synthetic materials release hundreds of volatile organic chemicals (VOCs) into the air. Over a period of many years Russian and American space scientists established that, in addition to carbon dioxide, we release as many as 150 volatile substances (bioeffluents) in the atmosphere, such as carbon monoxide, hydrogen, methane, alcohols, phenols, methyl indole, aldehydes, ammonia, etc. A number of illnesses have arisen from this indoor air pollution.[190]

In 1989 the EPA submitted a report to the U.S. Congress: "...sufficient evidence exists to conclude that indoor air pollution represents a major portion of the public's exposure to air pollution and may pose serious acute and chronic health risk." To sum up, three primary sources of poor indoor air quality are: hermetically sealed buildings and their synthetic furnishings, reduced ventilation, and human bioeffluents. On top of those add carbon dioxide from breathing.[191]

The National Aeronautics and Space Administration (NASA), faced with the task of creating a life-support system for planned moon bases, began extensive studies on treating and recycling air and wastewater. These studies led NASA scientists to ask a very important question. How does the earth produce and sustain clean air? The answer, of course, is through the living process of plants. Pollutants in the air are absorbed through microscopic openings in leaves called stomata and oxygen and water are released into the atmosphere. The pollutants are transported to the root zone and root microbes (i.e. pseudomonas) biodegrade the pollutants into structures that can be used as a source of food for the microbes and the plant. Hooray for the plants who help save the earth and give us oxygen![192]

People with any kind of degenerative disease would get better faster and easier if they were breathing clean air. The moral of this story is to have plants all around your house especially in the bedroom and the living room where you spend the most time.

Cancer grows in an aerobic condition, without oxygen. By having extra oxygen in the body will help to kill the cancer. Exercise also helps to breath in more oxygen. Another way is using an oxygen machine once or twice a day, which gives off pure oxygen, is best. But there is a difference between O_2 and O_3 for oxygen therapy. The stable O_2 that is in the air we breathe, along with O_3 gives us life but O_3 is what is really needed for oxygen therapy for degenerative diseases especially for cancer.

This protocol with its fasting and diet is high in antioxidents and is oxygen therapy itself but regular oxygen therapy would be very helpful in choking cancer to death! Cancer is anaerobic, it does not breath oxygen to live and when oxygen surrounds the cancer it chokes and dies! Technically the cancer cell starts to oxidize and break down the cancer. This also happens with other degenerative diseases.

C. Green Teas

Green tea is a very popular tea in Asia. Green tea is unfermented while black tea is fermented. The potency of the green tea can depend on the source, there are many sources.

Japanese have the highest smoking rate yet the lowest lung cancer rates in the world, they have one third lung cancer rates of American counterparts. In the 1980's Japanese researchers discovered the chemical in green tea that inhibited the growth of cancer: epigallocatechin gallate (EGCG).[193] It was shown to be able to inhibit tumor growth in the skin and gastrointestinal tract of experimental mice.[194] [195]

Dr. Hirota Fujiki of the National Cancer Center Research Institute in Tokyo stated: "We think that EGCG is the practical cancer chemo preventive agent to be implemented in everyday life." "Green tea cannot prevent every cancer, but it's the cheapest and most practical method for cancer prevention available to the general public."[196] EGCG could be a 'free radical scavenger,' neutralizing the highly reactive molecules that attack DNA and trigger cancer.

At the Rutgers University Laboratory for Cancer Research, Dr. Chung S. Yang and his colleagues found that green tea "significantly inhibited" stomach and lung cancer. The mice that drank the green tea had their tumors reduced by 60 to 63 percent.[197]

Chapter VI

Green CAM Nutrition Therapy

A. CAM and Green Paradigms

Chlorophyll rich foods were a basic clinical approach to medicine 100 years ago but then the pharmaceutical drug approach started to gain importance. A movement away from green foods and chlorophyll as a medical therapy started to take place. The allopathic medical paradigm emphasizing pharmaceutical drugs started to become the dominant player in medicine over the last 50 years.

There is a need to look at some basic medical paradigms as to why smoothies work for medical issues and curing illnesses and degenerative diseases. CAM means Complementary and Alternative Medicine and is an accepted approach in the U.S. and around the world. Green smoothies are a way to optimize the body and help improve or even help cure many health issues. Green Smoothies and Juicing can be a formal part of any CAM program for health and healing. To give some background on this topic will be helpful. We need to move towards green medical paradigms and Green Complementary and Alternative Medicine

Modern medicine and the pharmaceutical industry has only been around for less than a hundred years. Healing illness and degenerative diseases through nutrition and fasting or other detoxification techniques has been around in established medical practice for well over 1,000 years in India and China. The use of diet and fasting goes back over 2,000 years in the Jewish and Christian traditions. In fact these methods tend to be more effective then modern medicine most of the time, especially for serious degenerative diseases.

Diet Therapy, fasting and nutrients are considered part of Complementary and Alternative Medicine (CAM). These used to be one of the main tools of physicians before the advent of modern pharmaceuticals, drugs and other forms of medicine, like radiation or chemotherapy. The most predominate and most successful diet therapy programs are those that are raw vegan, living foods programs. Green smoothies are part of the basic emphasis on vegan (no meat or animal products), and little to no cooking (raw) equals living foods. In many of the major health resorts/institutes in the U.S. and overseas some kind of living foods orientation is used in which anywhere from 80/20 to 100% raw living foods is emphasized depending on the place.

"In addition to its acceptance by public sources of information, CAM has also entered mainstream medicine in an unprecedented fashion. An Office of Alternative Medicine (OAM) was established at the National Institutes of Health by Congressional mandate in 1992, its stated purpose being to investigate unconventional medical practices. Currently, the OAM supports 16 CAM Research Centers. Most, including the Center for Alternative Medicine Research in Cancer at the University of Texas Health Science Center in Houston, are based at major universities. With OAM, the relevant NIH institute shares support of basic science as well as clinical research within its purview. In October, 1998, Congress elevated the Office of Alternative Medicine to the 'National Center for Complementary and Alternative Medicine,' appropriating $50 million for its support.

Another marker of mainstream acceptance is the emergence of medical school courses in complementary and alternative medicine. Elective courses in CAM and portions or required courses are taught in at least 75 medical schools in the United States. In addition, numerous hospitals and medical centers have developed research and clinical service programs in CAM. Cancer programs and also many comprehensive cancer centers have implemented or are creating CAM programs of varying complexity."[198]

"Almost all studies conducted to date of cancer patients and of the general public internationally show that those who seek CAM therapies tend to be female, better educated, of higher socioeconomic status, and younger than those who do not. There is some indication of a growth in CAM use by cancer patients in recent years; a secondary analysis of close to 3,000 American cancer patients estimates a 64% increase since 1997 [at year 2,000]."[199]

Dr. Sidney Baker, M.D., gives a good definition of the kind of medical approach that a healing diet emphasizes in 'individual-oriented medicine'. "There is only one immunology and there is only one biochemistry. There are, however, two camps in medicine. Disease-oriented medicine and individual-oriented medicine (Dr. Galland's 'patient-centered diagnosis' or Dr. Jeffrey Bland's 'functional medicine' are other terms for this approach.) do not differ on the current facts of biochemistry and immunology. The difference is entirely one of orientation. Disease-oriented medicine is directed to finding the generalized formulas from treating groups of people who resemble one another in certain symptomatic respects. Such an approach is indispensable to thoughtful medical practice.

"The Individual-oriented medicine approach is to find everything possible that can be done to optimize the heath of a given unique individual. Such an approach is also indispensable to thoughtful medical practice and it requires a disquieting degree of judgment to know what individual differences are significant enough to treat. As I said earlier, if you do enough tests you can find something wrong with just about anyone. This phrase goes to the core of the medical dichotomy. In one camp is the attitude that whatever is found wrong must rise above individuality to join a pattern linked to a group of people who all have 'the same thing.' In the other camp is the attitude that an effort should be made to harmonize a patient's chemistry when it is clearly abnormal even though the abnormality does not constitute a disease."[200]

A green smoothie approach is about this 'Patient-centered diagnosis' or 'Individual-oriented medicine' in order to optimize the body via the diet, fasting and nutrients. This type of functional medicine tries to optimize a person's biochemistry and gene structure. Naturopathic medicine, Ortho-molecular medicine and Ayurveda Medicine also try to optimize the body through natural means. Green smoothies and juicing are part of that natural means.

We need to understand what a paradigm is and how science is basically a relative framework that evolves in time, such as going from Newtonian physics to Einstein's relativistic physics. They are both true but involve different paradigms of physics. Or more recently going from analog to digital television, which is a major paradigm shift. Another one is going from the mechanical watch to the digital watch. The Swiss watch market owned over 80% of the mechanical watch market in the world, then they developed digital watches, yet all the Swiss watchmakers laughed at it and ignored it, but it was taken seriously by other businessmen and now the Swiss watch market owns less than 20% of the world's market and digital watches in other countries own over 80%! We are talking about going from a drug-based model to a plant-based model, two different paradigms.

Now let us look at biology we all know that there are different types of medical doctors: allopathic (MD, DO), chiropractic (DC), naturopathic (ND) and others which are found in the U.S. and overseas. Then there are other health practitioners' such as homeopathic (big in Europe) or Ayurvedic (serving India's billion people) or Chinese medicine. These are a totally different paradigm then the allopathic model which is 'Germ-theory' based.

In the U.S. and Europe these different models boil down to two basic modern medical paradigms one that was created in the 1800's. It was Louis Pasteur in the 1800's that came up with the 'Germ Theory'. Drugs are created to kill these germs and to do other biochemical changes. But technically a drug is by definition, 'a legal low level synthetic poison.' Synthetic Drugs can be patented, owned and sold by drug companies, who make upwards of 800% profit. It is the pharmaceutical drugs and methods which support this medical paradigm of the germ theory, their drugs kill the germs! The major obstacle to this approach is allopathic medicine is based on giving pharmaceutical drugs not green smoothies, juices and living foods!

Back in Louis Pasteur's time was another more prominent Professor of medicine, Antoine Bechamp who brought his theory of microzymas public or in modern biochemical terminology it would be called, biological transmutations or the "Biological Terrain Theory". The germs are biologically transformed by the intracellular environment or they die off. In this model germs are not bad things but misplaced biological entities which can be transformed back to being good guys or just killed off! Just like an acidic cellular environment (usually unhealthy) can be transformed to a healthy alkaline environment. This paradigm is well accepted in molecular chemistry where chemicals change back and forth. This is the foundation for most natural medicine approaches. Actually Ayurvedic medicine in India and Chinese medicine are over 1,000 years old and have this medical model integrated as part of their system. This is what fasting and living foods do and it is the 'real purpose' of nutrition therapy which is to help the body cure itself through its own biological transformation in the Biological Terrain. It is a total paradigm shift in medicine. So the Germ Theory (Allopathic medicine) is one medical approach and Biological Terrain Theory (most natural medicine methods) is the other medical approach. These are two of the major medical paradigms and juicing and smoothies fit into the Biological Terrain Theory.

B. Green Nutrition Therapy

A perfect example of a nutritional therapy program with greens and green drinks curing cancer is the Gerson Diet which is known for being used for cancer. The Gerson diet is a raw vegan diet with 6 glasses of green drinks and six glasses of carrot juice a day. Now that's a lot of juice!

The Gerson Institute in San Diego did a study back in 1988. They raised about half a million dollars and worked with the University of California at San Diego's Cancer Prevention and Control Program study. They compared 5 year melanoma survival rates of Gerson therapy patients to rates found in comparable, conventionally treated groups in the medical literature. The study examined 153 white adult cancer patients, 25- 72 years old, in various stages of melanoma. The study found the following:

- Of patients with Stages I and II melanoma (localized), 100% of Gerson therapy patients survived for 5 years, compared with 79% of patients receiving conventional treatment.
- Of patients with Stages IIIa melanoma (regionally metastasized), 82% of Gerson therapy patients were still alive at 5 years, compared with 39% of those conventionally treated.
- Of patients with Stages IIIa and IIIb melanoma (regionally metastasized), 70% of Gerson therapy patients were still alive at 5 years, compared with 41% of the conventionally treated patients.
- Of patients with Stage IVa melanoma, 39% of Gerson therapy patients survived for 5 years, compared with 6% of patients treated by conventional medicine.[201]

A second study showed even higher rates for those with surgery plus Gerson Diet Therapy for a five year survival rate, since about a third of Gerson-treated patients had surgeries as well;[202] for stage IIIa 39% versus 92%, and for stage IVa 6% versus 57%."

This research and other scholarship is cited in the book, *Starving Cancer to Death*, by Jim Tibbetts and Joseph Spaziani, M.D. the emphasis is on a raw vegan diet or Living Foods diet to starve cancer to death!

The use of chlorophyll rich foods is needed to help put them into remission. Some of the basic benefits of plant-based nutrition for Parkinson's and other brain diseases are:

➤ Anti-Oxidant and Anti-Inflammatory
➤ Anti-Protein aggregation
➤ Anti-Excitotoxicity
➤ Mitochondria Protectors
➤ Balanced pH and sodium-potassium cellular levels
➤ Reduced pathogenic microorganisms and fungi levels
➤ Supports Brain homeostasis
➤ Neuroprotection leading to neuroplasticity and finally to neuroregeneration."

A Living Foods diet or the raw vegan diet is beyond the basic vegetarian diet which contains many highly cooked foods with grains, which is part of the cause, this feeds the diseases of Parkinson's, MS, Alzheimer's, ALS and other neurological diseases.

In these books a simple there is a more sophisticated approach and also a simple version of the Living Foods nutritional therapy for treating these types of diseases. This is a comprehensive lifestyle program in a more simplified format as follows:

• An 85/15% raw vegan diet, usually one meal is a large salad; this is a 100% vegan, 85% raw plant-based foods which has less than 15% cooked foods.
• Six 8oz glasses of freshly-juiced carrot juice daily; freshly-juiced apple or cucumber juice may replace up to half of the carrot juice;
• Six teaspoons of a green powder like barley grass powder daily;

- Breakfast should be juice, a smoothie, some fruit, or a light meal Lunch and Dinner consists of two large raw vegan meals (one is a large salad);
- Vigorous walking or exercise at least ½ hour a day to help digestion; include some sunshine, fresh air and prayer daily. Finally, a weekly meeting with a health professional is needed to work through the issues, both past and present.

This is the nutritional therapy in a nutshell. If the simplified version needs some adjunct therapies, it stays basically the same and supplements and other things are added on.

Because of the difficulty of eating the amount of greens necessary to get the chlorophyll needed it is easier to take green powders. It is very difficult to eat as many greens as are needed and making green juices from fresh, ripe, raw, organic plants is difficult and expensive. The Gerson Institute makes 6 glasses of green drinks and 6 glasses of carrot juice a day for their patients, which are mostly cancer patients. You need an expensive juicer and a lot of time to put into all the work of making green juices. Therefore using green powders is the next best option, to colloidal liquid nutrients in a bottle or juiced. The two best green powders are wheat grass and barley grass; they are best because a lot of research has been done on them showing their therapeutic value. About three grams (one heaping teaspoon) of barley powder is the equivalent of about two handfuls, or 100 grams, of the fresh young barley leaves.

For a Green Therapeutic Approach with Plant-based Nutrition for most degenerative diseases is summarized:

Plant-based Nutrition
1. Animal fat intake and animal products need to be zero.
2. Junk foods need to be zero, avoiding the five whites: sugar, salt, white flour, milk, and the fat on meats (any animal products).

3. No grains or beans unless they are soaked and sprouted.
4. An 80/20 to 100% raw vegan diet is the basic diet.
5. Minimizing fruit in the beginning stages/months to reduce intake of sugar in order to minimize yeast (*Candida Albicans*) growth.

Fasting, Smoothies and Juicing
6. Fasting and detox methods catabolize unwanted cells and also normalize cells to ideal levels.
7. Green Smoothies daily are essential.
8. Juicing on a daily basis to avoid dehydration and provide nutrients.

Supplements - Six Sigma rotation methodology
9. A nutritional supplement regime as needed.
10. Protein powders
11. Green powders

Complementary Therapies - that influence physiology
12. An exercise and relaxation routine is needed.
13. Prayer and Meditation reduce stress.
14. Various other adjunct therapies, like massage.

Some of the foods to avoid include the categories:
- First category is: Cooked and Processed foods including, canned, micro-waved, refined, GMO foods and other highly processed foods.
- Second category is: all Animal Products, including animal flesh, dairy, and eggs.
- Third category is: Grain products and most grains such as wheat, barley, oats, corn, white potatoes, white rice, white flour, soy products and peanuts (except sprouted grain products).
- Fourth category is: Sweeteners: sugar, honey, artificial sweeteners, maple syrup, fructose, and maltose and others.
- Fifth category is: heated oils (except coconut oil).

Sixth category is: beverages including alcohol, coffee, caffeine, all soda and carbonated beverages, bottled pasteurized juices.

The author Jim Tibbetts has two diets or nutritional programs, the diets are two different developments of the same paradigm; "The Alleluia Diet" which has a spiritual component and psychological intervention. Most medical personal would not want to admit that a diet doesn't work biochemically because there are psychological problems that are interfering with it, (this theory goes back to the time of Sigmund Freud) or that the people need to pray to God. The Alleluia diet is basically the same as "Six Sigma Nutrition" which does not emphasize a spiritual dimension or the need for psychological intervention, it is a paradigm focused on the space-time-causality of modern science.

Six Sigma Nutrition is based on six sigma technology found in industries like manufacturing, it is the same diet as the Alleluia diet but without any spiritual and psychological angle, and with a clinical approach for doctors, nutritionists and others. Six Sigma Nutrition is the approach in the medical community for Alzheimer's, Parkinson's, MS, cancer and other degenerative diseases; it has a clinical emphasize in nutrition. It is designed for those in the health field as just a purely scientific methodology yet it can include some psychological issues.

Psychological intervention is often needed and spiritual or religious motivation is a very powerful additive to the mixture, and spiritual healing does have a reality all its own. Medical doctors don't like to add in spiritual material or prayer and besides insurance companies won't pay for it!

Chapter VII

The Raw Family Teachings
on Green Smoothies

A. The Raw Family and Green Smoothies

In 2003 I (Jim) went to Oregon and spent a week
studying with the Raw Family in their week long raw food
chef training course. It was a great learning experience about
raw foods. I have followed their growth and development
since then and recommend their materials to others. I
consider Victoria Boutenko to be one of my teachers in this
field of raw vegan nutrition.

The Raw Family are one of the most well known and
loved raw families in the U.S. They are pioneers in the raw
field. They came from Russia in 1989 and in January 1994
they became raw fooders. Victoria Boutenko, her husband
Igor, and their children Valya, and Sergei, were healed from
degenerative diseases in 1994. Victoria had arrhythmia, or
an irregular heartbeat, her legs were constantly swollen from
edema. Igor had progressive hyperthyroidism and chronic
rheumatoid arthritis. Valya was born with asthma and
allergies and would often cough heavily all through the night.
Sergei was diagnosed with juvenile type-1 diabetes. Victoria
switched the whole family to a raw food diet and within a
year they were all healed of their health issues. They have
numerous books and videos worth viewing.

Victoria and her family began giving talks and
demonstrations on raw foods around the country. Her books
and website became a buzz and well known. Her early book,
Green for Life was on the benefits of greens and green
smoothies. The book became a best seller and has been
translated into numerous languages. Victoria is the one who
primarily started the Green Smoothies revolution, many

others have jumped on the band wagon with their own books and teachings and their own "School of Thought on Smoothies" on the best way to make a green smoothie! Yet Victoria stands out as the "Queen of Green Smoothies!"

Victoria Boutenko's School of Thought on Green Smoothies is one of the most well known and most widely accepted approaches. Green smoothies have been around for a long time but Victoria Boutenko was really one of the personalities who made it known and loved across the U.S. and now around the world with her books and travels. The following is her basic teaching on green smoothies which can be found on her website: www.rawfamily.com

B. Ten Health Benefits of Green Smoothies or Ode to Green Smoothies

The, Ten Health Benefits of Green Smoothies or the Ode to Green Smoothies[203] is from the raw family's website (earlier website cir 2009): www.rawfamily.com   this is a great summary!

What do I mean by green smoothie? Here is one of my favorite recipes: 4 ripe pears, 1 bunch of parsley and 2 cups of water. Blended well. This smoothie looks very green, but it tastes like fruit. I enjoy green smoothies so much that I bought an extra blender and placed it in my office, so that I could make green smoothies throughout the day. More than half of all the food I've had in last several months have been green smoothies. I have so much more energy and clarity that I have removed green juices from my diet. (Juicing has been something that I've been doing regularly for years.) Green smoothies have numerous benefits for human health.

1. Green smoothies are very nutritious. The ratio in them is optimal for human consumption; about 60% ripe organic fruit mixed with about 40% organic greens.

2. Green smoothies are easy to digest. When blended well, most of the cells in the greens and fruits are ruptured, making the valuable nutrients easy for the body to assimilate. Green smoothies literally start to get absorbed in your mouth.

3. Green smoothies, as opposed to juices, are a complete food because they still have fiber. Consuming fiber is important for our elimination system.

4. Green smoothies belong to the most palatable dishes for all humans of all ages. With a ratio of fruits to veggies as 60:40 the fruit taste dominates the flavor, yet at the same time the greens balance out the sweetness of the fruit, adding a nice zest to it. People who eat a standard American diet enjoy the taste of green smoothies. They are usually quite surprised that something so green could taste so nice.

5. A molecule of chlorophyll closely resembles a molecule of human blood. According to teachings of Dr. Ann Wigmore, consuming chlorophyll is like receiving a healthy blood transfusion. Many people do not consume enough greens, even those who stay on a raw food diet. By drinking two or three cups of green smoothies daily you will consume enough greens for the day to nourish your body, and all of the beneficial nutrients will be well assimilated.

6. Green smoothies are easy to make, and quick to clean up after. In contrast, juicing greens is time consuming, messy, and expensive. Many people abandon drinking green juices on a regular basis for those reasons. To prepare a pitcher of green smoothie takes less than 5 minutes, including cleaning.

7. Green smoothies have proven to be loved by children of all ages, including babies of six or more months old. Of course you have to be careful and slowly increase the amount of smoothies to avoid food allergies.

8. When you consume your greens in the form of green smoothies, you can greatly reduce the consumption of oils and salt in your diet.

9. Regular consumption of green smoothies forms a good habit of eating greens. After a few weeks of drinking green smoothies, most people start to crave and enjoy eating more greens. Eating enough greens is often a problem with many people, especially children.

10. While fresh is always best, green smoothies will keep in cool temperatures for up to three days, which can be handy at work and while traveling.

Start playing with green smoothies, and discover the many joys and benefits of this wonderful delicious and nutritious addition to your menu.

C. Guidelines to Drinking Green Smoothies

This article (2009); Guidelines to Drinking Green Smoothies[204] is a must read for all green smoothie drinkers. Through everyday blending, research, experience, and letters from readers, the Raw Family has come up with these basic principles for green smoothie making and consuming. To help people receive the most benefits from drinking green smoothies and to avoid some typical mistakes, Victoria created the following guidelines:

- Prepare your green smoothie first thing in the morning in the amount that you usually consume in one day, one or two quarts (liters). Pour enough smoothie in a glass for your morning enjoyment and keep the rest in a refrigerator or another cold place.
- Sip your green smoothie slowly, mixing it with saliva. Sometimes I put my smoothie in a coffee mug with a lid and carry it with me to the car or to my office.

That way I minimize a chance of spilling it and keep it private without distracting others.

- Don't add anything to your smoothie except greens, fruit and water. I don't recommend adding nuts, seeds, oils, supplements or other ingredients to your green smoothie. Most of these items slow down the assimilation of green smoothies in your digestive tract and may cause irritation and gas. Even though I provide recipes with more than basic ingredients in my books I encourage you to stick to the basic green smoothie recipe (fruit and greens) in your daily routine.

- Drink your smoothie by itself, and not as a part of a meal. Don't consume anything, even as little as a cracker or candy with it. You may eat anything you want approximately 40 minutes before or 40 minutes after you finished your smoothie. Your goal is to get the most nutritional benefit out of your green smoothie.

- Do not add starchy vegetables such as carrots, beets, broccoli stems, zucchini, cauliflower, cabbage, Brussels sprouts, egg plant, pumpkin, squash, okra, peas, corn, green beans, and others to your green smoothies. Starchy vegetables combine poorly with fruit and may produce what my children call "gas 4 less."

- Don't add too many ingredients into one smoothie, such as nine different fruits and a dozen different greens. Try to keep most of your recipes simple to maximize nutritional benefits and to keep it easy on your digestive system.

- Learn to prepare a really delicious green smoothie so that you are always looking forward to the next one. If your drink is not tasty, you will eventually discontinue consuming it. Keep your taste buds happy.

- Always rotate the green leaves that you add to your smoothies. Almost all greens in the world contain minute amounts of alkaloids. Tiny quantities of alkaloids cannot hurt you, and even strengthen the immune system. However, if you keep consuming kale, or spinach, or any other single green for many weeks without rotation, eventually the same type of alkaloids can accumulate in your body and cause unwanted symptoms of poisoning. Please note that you don't have to rotate the fruit in your green smoothies. Most commonly used fruit have very little or none of the alkaloids and cannot cause the same toxic reactions as greens. At the same time, rotating fruits will enhance the variety of flavor and nutrition in your smoothies.

Choose organic produce whenever possible. The absence of pesticides and other toxic chemicals is only one of many benefits of organic food. The most important reason to consume organic food is the superior nutritional of organic fruits and vegetables in comparison to conventionally grown produce. We have been discussing earlier, how deficient most people are. The best way to nourish your body is to consume organic produce and whenever possible, locally grown. I consider it very important to get the fruit that was allowed to ripen on the vine because it is the best for nourishment. Tree-ripened fruit is several times more nutritious and when consumed shortly after picking retains significantly more nutrients.

D. Common Green Smoothie Questions
answered by Victoria

These Q&A are from Victoria's Raw Family's website (2009).[205]

QUESTION: Do I have to make fresh smoothie several time per day?

VICTORIA: Smoothies can stay in the refrigerator for 2-3 days, but fresh is best. As soon as a smoothie is warmed to room temperature, it should be consumed.

QUESTION: How much green smoothie do you recommend I drink daily?

VICTORIA: In the beginning people tend to drink more green smoothies, sometimes up to two gallons per day depending on how acidic their body pH is. After several months the quantity goes down to 1-2 quarts per day.

QUESTION: I have been on raw food for eight years and feel that my body is very clean. Why do I feel nauseous from drinking wheatgrass juice?

VICTORIA: If you have read my book *Green for Life*, you are familiar with the part where I speak about all greens, without exception, containing alkaloids. Alkaloid build up is toxic. Wheatgrass also contains a small amount of alkaloids. If you begin to drink it on a regular basis, the alkaloids accumulate and the body rejects it. This is why people get nauseous after drinking wheatgrass regularly for a while. When they take a break and come back to it, they can tolerate it better. Many people do not consume enough greens, and due to the fact that wheatgrass juice is almost 100% chlorophyll, the benefits of chlorophyll override the drawback of poisoning by alkaloids. That means, that even though people still get the alkaloid poisoning, the presence of chlorophyll in their body still helps to heal cancer, makes the body more alkaline and has other healing effects. That is why the green smoothies are so helpful, because when one begins to use a larger variety of greens in the form of green smoothies, one doesn't have to constantly drink wheatgrass juice. Just keep rotating and get as many different greens as you can.

QUESTION: I tested my urine and my saliva. My urine is very alkaline and my saliva is very acidic. I think I am still detoxing (four weeks raw now) because I have cold sores, rashes etc. Could that be why my saliva is acidic or is it not a good way to judge your PH level? I just don't understand why they are both so completely different.

VICTORIA: Measuring your body pH by testing your urine is much more accurate than testing saliva. Alkalinity in saliva appears only after having the body's alkaline pH established for some time. Also, saliva changes more rapidly and more often than urine. You can do some experimenting: for example if you put a drop of honey on your tongue, the saliva instantly becomes very alkaline because the alkaline solution amylase (that helps digests sugar) will be present in the saliva. If you put a teaspoon of any green smoothie or wheatgrass in your mouth, your saliva instantly becomes acid, because in order to digest greens, the saliva first has to become acid. Of course, greens are alkaline-forming once digested. So, testing pH by checking saliva is tricky. It has to be a long time between meals, you have to have your mouth clean and empty, and not even have food in SIGHT. That is why I don't recommend it. Urine doesn't change by what we look at, and thus is more reliable. The most accurate time to test saliva for alkalinity is in the morning as soon as you wake up.

QUESTION: I drove to three towns, at least eighty miles apart from each other and looked in more than five different health food stores. When I asked the produce person for lambsquarters, plantain, chickweed, stinging nettles, purslane, etc., they looked at me like I was nuts! For lambsquarters, they kept sending me to the meat department. Where and how can one find the wild edible greens?

VICTORIA: Even though it can be difficult for one to buy wild edible greens in the store, one still would greatly benefit from consuming them. That is why I put wild edible greens in my smoothie recipes.

I don't have a way of recommending which wild plants are edible in your area since I am unsure of what weeds grow in your area. The best thing to do is to talk to people who plant flowers and bushes in parks. They can usually identify edible plants quite well. Another way to find out which plants one can eat is to talk to farmers, who need help weeding their organic gardens. In the summer, my children pick lambsquarters and plantain from a local farmer who pays them to pluck these pesky weeds from his fields. Once you learn to recognize a couple of edible weeds, it's a good idea to share your knowledge with others so that you can learn about sill more scrumptious plants. This year, I plan to plant lots weeds in my own garden. I will report back to you how that works out for me.

QUESTION: Do you think it is beneficial or helpful to add any fat to raw smoothies? I don't eat salads, so instead I just add a little fat, a couple tablespoons of flax seeds, or half an avocado, occasionally I will have a whole one if I'm feeling really decadent.

VICTORIA: Each person is unique and thus has different needs. Some people might need fat, however, fat does slow down the digestive process. You may add anything you want to your smoothie to make it suit your personal needs. As for me, I believe that Green Smoothies are a complete food.

QUESTION: Do you think it is better to use powdered greens in green smoothies as opposed to fresh greens?

VICTORIA: I think that if one remembers to rotate the greens they consume and drink at least one quart of green smoothie per day, they will receive an optimal amount of nutrients. I recommend leaving green powders for the times when green smoothies are not accessible for example, during travels. I do not think that dried greens are nearly as vibrant or nutritious as fresh greens. My daughter Valya recently decided to further explore the theory of dried versus fresh greens with a group of volunteers who were not susceptible to advertisements. It happened that my husband was invited to help out at a horse farm. Valya preformed an experiment by offering six horses the option eating green, professionally dried, high quality hay, (super food) or fresh kale, and grass. Six out of six horses chose the fresh greens over the dry hay. (Heh-heh...)

QUESTION: How many greens does one really need? I generally consume a head of lettuce. Do you think this is enough?

VICTORIA: One needs fewer greens in the form of green smoothies than in the form of salad, because blended greens assimilate several times more thoroughly then chewed greens. People who have an acidic pH balance in their body could benefit from consuming up to 80% greens in their diet. When they reach a stage of balance, they will notice that they want less greens and less green smoothies, but they will enjoy them more than ever.

QUESTION: When greens are broken up in the blender, do they oxidize and lose most of their nutrients? Incidentally, I do consume a ton of greens by eating huge salads and juicing.

VICTORIA: In my book, *Green For Life*, I explain that in order to get nutrients from greens, every cell of the green leaf has to be ruptured. To get all of the nutrients from food by oral mastication, one would have to spend several hours a day chewing, and have extremely healthy teeth that are all in place, including wisdom teeth. By observing the results of

those who regularly consume green smoothies, I now think
that the assimilation of nutrients from smoothies is several
times more efficient than from chewing greens. Of course,
these numbers are different from person to person, but I
estimate that two bunches of greens chewed are equal to
approximately to half a bunch of greens blended (not juiced,
because juice is missing an important ingredient: fiber).
When I was juicing my greens on a daily basis, I noticed how
quickly the green juice turned brown and began to taste
bitter. This doesn't appear to happen with blended greens,
probably because of the large quantities of antioxidants in the
fiber. Green smoothies continue to stay bright green and
taste fresh for many hours if kept in a cool place.

QUESTION: I thought Victoria's point for green smoothies
being superior to green juices was lacking. One of the main
benefits of juice is that it requires next to no digestion and
can be absorbed and assimilated immediately into the
bloodstream, allowing the digestive system to rest.

VICTORIA: I agree with Dr. Doug Graham that juices are a
fractured food, which is missing an essential component—
fiber. I believe that when we consume enough fiber, we take
a load off of our organism by dramatically improving our
elimination. Toxins build up in the colon. Fiber cleans them
out. When most toxins have been removed by fiber, then the
body has a greater ability to absorb nutrients, thus improving
digestion. There are many more important benefits in having
fiber. For example, in my previous newsletter, I cited
research about good bacteria needing raw fiber from fruits
and vegetables in our colon to be able to survive. These
bacteria are linked to the B complex vitamins--another
important issue. Juices are not a complete food; humans
could not live on juices alone. Very often juices have
unbalanced amounts of sugar. Contrary to juices, green
smoothies are a complete food. Also, I have met people who
went on prolonged juice fasts and saw no improvement in
their hydrochloric acid.

E. Stomach Acid and Raw Foods

Hydrochloric acid in the stomach is important to human health. When the human body is unable to produce enough stomach acid the condition of low stomach acidity (hypochlorhydria) occurs. This impacts the digestion and absorption of many nutrients and can lead to nutritional deficiencies and this could develop into diseases. When pathogenic bacteria, parasites, harmful microorganisms and fungi can enter the body through the mouth and if the stomach acid is insufficient then there is no barrier against these organisms.

Professor W. A. Walker from the Department of Nutrition at Harvard School of Public Health, states that, "Medical researchers since the 1930's have been concerned about the consequences of hypochlorhydria. While all the health consequences are still not entirely clear, some have been well documented."[206] Hypochlorhydria is low stomach acidity, when the body is not producing enough stomach acid. This impacts digestion and absorption of nutrients. Stomach acid also destroys all harmful microorganisms, pathogenic bacteria, parasites and their eggs, and fungi that enter the body through the mouth. "Stomach acid helps to digest large protein molecule.[207]

As we age, especially after 40, the level of hydrochloric acid (HCL) decreases. If we abuse our body through excess food and the wrong types of foods it can also cause the hydrochloric acid to decrease. "Overeating, especially over consumption of fats and proteins, wears out the parietal cells of the stomach that secret HCL."[208] "Stomach acid helps to digest large protein molecules. If stomach acid is low, then incompletely digested protein fragments get absorbed into the bloodstream and cause allergies and immunological disorders."[209]

Blending foods is similar to chewing foods; unfortunately most people do not chew their foods enough to break them down completely. A high speed blender breaks the foods down for easier assimilation. The food doesn't stay in the stomach as long so less hydrochloric acid is needed. Thus the process of blending helps the body out in terms of not needing to produce more HCL, saves energy, and easier assimilation.

One of the problems on the raw food diet is that some people lose weight and stay thin as raw fooders being considered skinny. "For many years I couldn't understand why some people quickly loose too much weight on a raw food diet. These people simple cannot stay on a raw food diet because they feel uncomfortable living their lives with constant remarks from their friends and relatives about being too thin. I agree that humans shouldn't be too skinny."

Victoria Boutenko noticed this and did a lot of research about the impact of hypochlorhydria on assimilation of food. She found that some of her friends were diagnosed with very low or no stomach acid at all and their doctors prescribed HCL pills to take with their meals. One of her close friends was diagnosed with achlorhydria (no stomach acid) and was put on HCL pills. She continued on her raw food diet and gained back all her weight. "A close friend has been trying to eat raw for several years and became so thin that her husband became concerned for her health. She went to a doctor and was diagnosed with achlorhydria (no stomach acid). Her doctor put her on HCL pills and she continued her raw food diet. My friend gained all her weight back."[210]

The tough cellulose structure for most vegetables and some fruits needs to be ruptured to get all the nutrients out of the cells. Foods need stomach acids to help break down these cell walls. If there is not enough stomach acid then the body will not be able to receive all of these nutrients appropriately. These raw nutrients are a major benefit that is often lost in cooked foods. Deficiencies and degenerative diseases can

89

start to develop without these nutrients. Some people when eating raw foods were able to eliminate these symptoms of various illnesses but they became skinny. Then they would add cooked foods to their diet and they would gain weight but their unwanted symptoms would return. Victoria noted that:

"Puzzled, they kept going back and forth no knowing what to do. That is why I felt great joy when, after teaching a couple of classes about green smoothies, I began receiving letters like this one:

Though the raw food took care of my arthritis I was never able to stick to it longer than two months because on raw foods alone, I dropped weight so quickly, down to 135 lbs, that my wife panicked thinking I was dying, so I had to go back to cooked foods which made my arthritis return. When I started drinking green smoothies, my weight stabilized! I have been raw now for six months and keep my normal weight of 155 lbs. Thanks you!" (N.H., Canada)

I have already witnessed many cases in which people with digestive problems were able to greatly improve their assimilation by adding blended greens to their diets. While cooking makes the food softer and easier to digest, in the process of heating, most essential vitamins and enzymes in the food does get destroyed. Blending is a lot less harmful than cooking because it saves all the vital nutrients in the food."

"There are numerous conditions that are associated with low stomach acidity.[211] These are just some of them: bacterial overgrowth, chronic candidacies, parasites, Addison's disease, multiple sclerosis, arthritis, asthma, auto immune disorders, celiac disease, stomach carcinoma, depression, dermatitis, diabetes, eczema, flatulence, gall bladder disease, gastric polyps, gastritis, hepatitis, hyperthyroidism, myasthenia gravis, osteoporosis, psoriasis, rosacea, ulcerative colitis, urticaria, and vitiligo.

"That is why the famous researcher, Dr. Theodore A. Baroody, stated in his wonderful book *Alkalize or Die*, 'Hydrochloric acid is absolutely essential for life.' In other words, no one can be completely healthy without normal hydrochloric acid. 'Hydrochloric acid is the only acid that our body produces. All other acids are by-products of metabolism and are eliminated as soon as possible.'"[212]

F. The Roseburg Green Smoothie Study

Victoria Boutenko was interested in doing a study on the effects of green smoothies on stomach acid. She wanted to find several people who were diagnosed with low hydrochloric acid and would add green smoothies to their diets to see if it helped. She was praying to find a doctor who would be willing to help with the study and one morning a physician named Dr. Paul Fieber called from Roseburg in Oregon. Victoria wrote, "By some magical coincidence," they had recently adopted a raw food lifestyle and he was concerned about the number of people with low stomach acid. He agreed to assist and be involved in a study and the next week 85 people came for a nutrition class by Victoria and 27 people stepped forward and volunteered for the study. The study involved drinking one quart of freshly made smoothies each day while they continued to eat their standard American diet.

For the whole month of May the raw family blended many gallons of green smoothies and they drove 240 miles round trip, every other day to Roseburg from Ashland, Oregon to drop off the green smoothies. Every one of the participants came to pick up the smoothies throughout the study. Dr. Paul Fieber used the HCL challenge test to test each individual's pH levels. This test is designed to help determine the ability of the stomach to produce adequate stomach acid.

Many people have a deficient acid-producing process and suffer from hypochlorhydria and others have gastric reflux due to "excess" stomach acid secretions. For this excess antacid therapy has nothing to do with a cure and only provides temporary relief. Out of 27 participants only 2 people dropped out because they had no hypochlorhydria and the rest who participated all had some degree of hypochlorhydria. The ages ranged from 17 to 80. All the participants were asked not to change any other part of their diet except to drink the green smoothies, but after the study many did.

"After 30 days of drinking one quart of green smoothie each day, we then completed another HCL challenge test to see what improvement occurred over the month. One person dropped out in the middle of the study due to nausea. Out of the 24 participants we had only 16 of the group who showed improvement in their production of HCL. It was remarkable to me that 66.7% of the participants showed such vast improvement. I did not expect to see this much progress in such a short period of time. The fiber content and nutrient value of the green smoothies made for an incredible success. All the participants also noted many other improvements in their health, some of which were dramatic changes.

I would like to give my own personal testimonial as my wife and I had been drinking the green smoothies about two months before the study was conducted. My blood pressure, pulse rate, and cholesterol readings all improved substantially. We lost all cravings for cooked food and the green smoothies were both delicious and fulfilling. The most significant change for me concerned a small growth that had appeared on m nose. After one month on the green smoothies, the growth fell off and left a small hole where it once was. This proved to me the tremendous healing properties of green smoothie."[213] (Citing: Dr. Paul Fieber)

"As a result of regular consumption of the green smoothies for just one month, people named the following improvements: increase in energy, depression lifted and all suicidal thoughts gone, less blood sugar fluctuations, more regular bowel movements, dandruff healed, insomnia gone, asthma attacks stopped completely, none of usual 'PMS' symptoms any more, fingernails became stronger, wanted less coffee, sex life improved, skin cleared up, and many more. It was interesting to see that most of the participants who wanted to lose weight lost anywhere from five to ten pounds, and a couple of people who wanted to gain weight, were able to gain one or two pounds."[214]

The following chart is based on the "Raw Data" that Victoria gave in her book. She asked each of the participants 12 questions and they each answered them. If they did not answer a question it was filed under 'No comment'. Victoria gave the answers for each of the participants in a raw, unedited form. From this raw data the answers could be categorized into three broad possibilities. The three types of answers were a "Yes with a positive experience," or a "Yes with a negative experience" or a "No" or a No comment. For the complete set of 24 testimonials see Victoria's book *Green for Life*. It is obvious from looking at the chart it was an overall positive experience for everyone.

Raw Data for the Roseburg Study

Yes Positive   = Yes Pos.
Yes Negative = Yes Neg.
No Comment = No Com.

	Yes Pos.	Yes Neg	No	No Com	% of Positive Change
1. Was it hard to	1	2	20	1	20/23 =

drink one quart of Green Smoothie every day?					87%
2. Did the rest of your diet change as a result of the green smoothies?	19		1	4	19/20 = 95%
3. Did you notice any change in your health?	21		1	2	21/22 = 95%
4. Did your cravings for unhealthy foods lessen?	20		1	3	20/21 = 96%
5. Have you noticed any change in your weight?	16		4	4	16/20 = 80%
6. Did your sleep change?	19		1	4	19/20 = 95%
7. Did your elimination change?	20			4	20/20 = 100%
8. Did your energy change?	18		3	3	18/21 = 86%
9. Did anybody comment on how you looked?	8		5	9	8/13 = 62% *
10. Did you have any symptoms of detox?	3	11	6	4	14/20 = 70% **
11. Did you have any negative experiences?	1	1	18	4	18/20 = 90%
12. Would you like to continue drinking Green Smoothies?	22			2	22/22 = 100%

	Yes Pos	Yes Neg	No	No Com	92.4% Positive

* Commenting on how one looks is not in the same category of internal physical experiences since it is a social aspect and thus does not belong in the total average %.
** The negative experience of detox is actually a good thing and positive for helping to improve the physiological aspect.
*** Eight of the twelve questions have a 90% or above and the overall average positive score for 24 people for all the categories (except #9)* is over 90%. The no comments were not figured into the average score which is actually 90.4%. The only question that rated low was the detox symptoms question. This question actually skewed the % lower and without it the average positive score would be 92.4%

As can be seen from the chart the overall experience is positive for the individuals and more than 92% had a positive experience and benefit to their health in the categories! With these positive figures we can shout, Alleluia! This is the Alleluia Green Zone!

Some examples of the answers on this study are below which gives an indication of the positive effects green smoothies were having on the people. The no answers were mostly a positive. The Yes negative were primarily for the symptoms of detox which they had and were negative in the sense of the symptoms. But detox is actually a very positive house cleaning of the body which was getting rid of toxins and poisons. This gives an insight into the answers. For complete answers see the book; *Green for Life* by Victoria Boutenko. Below is the summary of comments.

Questions for Roseburg Study
1. Was it hard to drink one quart of Green Smoothie every day?
2. Did the rest of your diet change as a result of the green smoothies?
3. Did you notice any changes in your health?
4. Did your cravings for unhealthy foods lessen?
5. Have you noticed any change in your weight?
6. Did your sleep change?
7. Did your elimination change?
8. Did your energy change?
9. Did anybody comment on how you looked?
10. Did you have any symptoms of detox?

11. Did you have any negative experiences?

12. Would you like to continue drinking Green Smoothies?

Summary of Comments on Study by Participants

Yes positive – answers:

1. I wish I could have more a day;

2. Made more smoothies and ate less desserts; I stopped craving sugars and carbohydrates; Eating all raw;

3. More energy and weight loss; I require less sleep, my temperament is more even and pleasant; Ability to run longer without being out of breath; Less asthma; Yes, I have more energy and my husband is easier to get along with; I noticed an improvement in my skin – especially on days when I did not eat other junk;

4. I am not craving junk! Less ice cream these days; Yes, desire less chocolate and sweets at work; My cravings are almost gone for alcohol, sweets and chocolate! Thank goodness!; Yes, I eat far less junk;

5. Lost 4-5 lbs.; Lost 9-11 lbs.; I've lost 5-6 lbs.; Yes. 3 lbs. weight loss; I have lost 18-20 lbs.; Yes, I lost 10 lbs.;

6. I sleep sounder; My sleep is much better; Sleep better and a deeper sleep; Sleeping deeper, dreaming for the first time in almost a year;

7. Definitely regular. My bowel movement is great now!; More frequent;

8. Yes, I have a lot more energy; increased sex drive;

9. Yes, glowing; One person said I looked good; I was told I was glowing. Sex life improved; Yes, said I looked less stressed; I did have a couple of mild compliments;

10. Irregular itching all over my body during the first week; Slight nausea or heartburn; Only the mild detox; Spots like pimples or rash (not hives);

11. No negatives;

12. Yes, absolutely positive; Plant to do so! Great sex; I'm calmer, more peaceful, less anxious; Yes, I want to keep it up;

Yes negative – answers

1. At first. ; 2. --- ; 3. --- ; 4. --- ; 5. --- ; 6. --- ; 7. --- ; 8. --- ; 9. ---

10. Yes, stomach cramps and bloated first couple days; Some, headache, more acne; mild headaches; I did have mild mucus coughing and through sinuses, also mild nausea the first few days; I had detox headaches for a night and a day; 11. Only a mild detox; None; 12. ---

No – answers

1. No, however I wouldn't want more; No – sometimes I wanted more; No, not at all – I could drink them all day long;

2. No. I think I crave sugar a little less; It was easy and enjoyable. More would have been nice; 3. No. My weight is yo-yoing. 4. No.

5. No weight change. Never has been; No, stayed the same; 6. No. 7.---

8. Didn't notice any energy change;

9. No one commented; Not to my face anyway;

10. No symptoms that I felt; No bad reactions whatsoever;

11. None at all; No – It was very positive; No negative experiences; Nothing negative; 12. ---

Chapter VIII

Green Food Smoothie Creations

A person can start with a green drink, then they can make it into a green smoothie, then they can make that into a smoothie pudding, then they can make it into a smoothie soup, then they can make it into a salad smoothie and finally they can turn it into a Paté Short Soup. Another approach is to sit down to dinner with a green smoothie for a drink, a green smoothie soup to start with, then have a green smoothie salad, for dinner have a green Paté and green Paté Short Soup, and close with a green smoothie pudding! This chapter will show you the way to do all this - green! A little green humor is always helpful at times! But of course if you choose to start with a beet then everything would be red instead!   A rainbow of green benefits!

A. Green Smoothie's

Two basic ways to make a smoothie:
1. Build your own smoothie.
2. Follow the smoothie recipes in this book.

The long term goal is for people to be able to create their own smoothie from what they have available and get into the habit of buying the stuff that you need to make the smoothies so you have it. But giving recipes helps in starting out and helps with ideas that we may not have thought of on our own.

To build your own smoothie has several steps which involve choosing a **base** (fruit and/or vegetable), choosing the liquid **blend** and then choosing the **boosters**.

1. Choose your **Vegetable Base**, examples;
   - Spinach
   - Kale
   - Cucumber
   - Beet
   - Other vegetables

2. Choose your **Fruit Base**, examples;
   - Banana
   - Mango
   - Berries
   - Apples
   - Other fruits

3. Choose your **Liquid Blend**;
   - Water
   - Fruits juices
   - Vegetable juices
   - Coconut water
   - Other liquids such as tea

4. Choose your **Boosters**, examples;
   - Protein powders
   - Green powder
   - Flax oil
   - Honey
   - Bee pollen
   - Wheat germ
   - Other boosters

A smoothie is a mixture of a fruit or vegetable mix that is thin enough to drink. If it gets to thick like a pudding then just add more water. All smoothies can be made into pudding by adding less water or by adding a thickener, like nuts or seeds. Usually it can be easiest to start with softer produce and liquid then add harder fruits or veggies later. Always keep some fruits at home, it can be cut in chunks and in the freezer ready to use. Some of the fruit in freezer sections may not be organic but it is at least without preservatives or additives.

The following Smoothies are examples of building your own smoothie. Almost every one of these smoothies was made with the ingredients that was available in the kitchen at the time that they were made. Of course during shopping we realize that we will be making smoothies and but fruits and vegetables for the smoothie and to eat.

a. Jim's Smoothie Creations

The following are some smoothie creations by the author. These were all tried out but some of Jim's creations may need more sweetness or other items added or deleted. You'll have to decide. Come up with your own creations!

A Smashing Smoothie	Red Berry Smoothie
1 – small apple Handful – spinach ½ - cup carrot juice Slice – red cabbage	½ - cup berry juice 1 – tomato 1 handful – baby spinach
Jazzman Smoothie	**Red Sunset**
1 – cup apple juice ½ - cup blueberries ½ - cucumber 2 – broccoli trees ½ - teaspoon flax oil	1 – cup tomato juice 1 – cucumber ½ handful lettuce 1-2 - broccoli trees 1 tbsp – protein powder

Rock n'Roll Smoothie ½ cup – juice mixture one or more of the following: (blueberry, blackberry, grape, or other juices) 1 – cucumber 1 ½ - sticks celery 1 handful – spinach 1 scoop protein powder	**Blue Moon** 1 – cup water 1 – cup blueberries Handful baby spinach Small slice onion 1 tbsp – flax oil 1 tbsp – protein powder
Pine Spin Cuke 2 cups pineapple juice 1 orange 2 handfuls of spinach 1 apple 1 cucumber 1 cup water 1 scoop protein powder 1 tbsp maca powder 1 tbsp bee pollen 1tbsp Udo's oil	**Hopping Rabbit** Several Sections of fennel ¼ cup of parsley 2 leaves of lettuce ½ cucumber 2 stalks of celery ¼ orange pepper Dash sea salt or unrefined salt (optional) 1 scoop protein powder (optional) 1 tbsp honey (optional)
Coconut Green Swinger 1 – cup coconut juice 1 - 2 cups spinach 1 tbsp – protein powder	**Chinatown** 1 cup – hot miso soup reconstitute (powder form or live) 1 – stalk celery ¼ - yellow pepper 2 -3 broccoli trees ½ - peeled cucumber 1 – scoop protein powder

Power Punch Smoothie 1 cup water Handful lettuce 1 banana ½ cucumber 1 scoop Protein powder (optional) 1 tablespoon *Udo's Oil* (optional) 1 teaspoon green powder (optional)	**Daisy Duck Smoothie** 1 cup water ½ cucumber Several sections fennel 2 -3 leaves lettuce ½ handful parsley Slice orange pepper 1scoop protein powder (optional) 1 tbsp green powder (optional)
Scoop of Fun 2 cups any fruit 2 cups any veggie 1 cup any juice 1 cup water 1 scoop protein powder 1 scoop of fun!	**Space Walk Smoothie** 1 cup water 2 - 3 broccoli tops 2 leaves lettuce 1 peeled carrot Several sections of fennel ¼ cup parsley 1 small piece green onion
Veggie Tango 1 banana ¼ cup parsley Handful spinach 1 -2 stalks celery 1 cup water 1 scoop protein powder	**Orange Rain** Juice of 1 orange ½ peeled cucumber 1 banana ½ cup water 2 - 3 leaves lettuce 1 scoop protein powder

Pineapple Cuke	Mango Spinach
1 peeled cucumber 1 cup pineapple 1 banana 1 large leaf Swiss chard ½ cup water	1 mango 1 handful spinach 1 banana ½ peeled cucumber ½ cup water
Broccoli Cuke 1 peeled cucumber 1 handful spinach 2 -3 broccoli trees ½ cup fruit juice blend 1 scoop protein powder (optional)	**Tomato Cuke** 1 banana ½ peeled cucumber ½ tomato ¼ cup cilantro ¼ cup parsley ½ cup water 1 scoop protein powder
I Dreamed of Veggies 2 small carrots 1 piece cauliflower 4 pieces asparagus 2 broccoli trees 1 sections of leek 1 cup water 1 scoop protein powder	**Mountain-view** 1 – cup water 1 – tomato Juice of 1 lemon ½ - peeled cucumber 1 -2 leaves of lettuce 2 broccoli trees Pinch of kelp granules
Veggie Melody 1 – cup water 2 cups of the following vegetables chopped and mixed for a salad: Peeled Carrots Beets Celery Peeled Cucumber	**Berry Overture** 1 cup water 1 ½ cups frozen berries 1 banana 3 tbsp cocoa powder (optional) 1 tbsp green barley 2 tbsp Chia seeds, soaked for 1 hour

Red cabbage Cauliflower Broccoli Onion Tomato Lettuce Orange pepper	1 cup coconut water 1 scoop hemp protein (optional) 1 tbsp honey 1 tbsp coconut oil
Blue Cuke Cado 1 avocado 1 cup blueberries 1 banana 1 cucumber 1 handful spinach 1 cup pineapple juice 1 cup water 1 tbsp Udo's oil 1 scoop protein powder 1 tbsp bee pollen	**Pine Cuke Spin** 1 banana 1 cucumber 1 handful spinach 1 apple 1 cup pineapple juice 1 cup water 1 tbsp Udo's oil 1 scoop protein powder 1 tbsp bee pollen
Honey Melon Mango ½ honey dew melon 1 banana 1 avocado 2 C. baby spinach 1 cup mango nectar 1 C. berry veggie juice blend 2 cups water 1 scoop protein powder	**Car-Cel-Cuc Berry** 1 cup carrot juice ½ cup celery juice ½ cup cucumber juice Berry smoothie drink Bunch spinach Few pieces broccoli 1 banana 1 scoop protein powder 1 teaspoon Udo's oil 1 teaspoon almond butter

b. The Raw Family Green Smoothies

These are some Green Smoothie Recipes by the Raw Family - these and others are on their website (2009) and designated as free to use.[215]   (www.rawfamily.com)

Apple-kale-lemon	Peach-spinach
4 apples ½ lemon juice 5 leaves of kale 2 cups water	6 peaches 2 handfuls of spinach leaves 2 cups water
Mango-weeds 2 mangos 1 handful of edible weeds, such as lambsquarters, stinging nettles, purslane, etc 2 cups water	**Orange, Yellow, and Green Smoothie** 1 bunch spinach 2 oranges (peeled with seeds removed) ¼ lemon with peel (seeds removed) 4 dates (with pits removed) 2 frozen bananas 2 cups water ¼ teaspoon nutmeg
Strawberry-banana-romaine smoothie 1-cup strawberries 2 bananas ½ bunch romaine 2 cups water	**Pear-kale-mint smoothie** 4 ripe pears 5 leaves of kale ½ bunch of mint 2 cups water
Basic Balance *Victoria Boutenko* 1 mango 1 cup kale 1 cup water	**Victoria's Favorite Dark Green** *Victoria Boutenko* 1 bunch dandelion greens 4 Roma tomatoes

	3 cups water
Yields 1 quart	Yields 2 quarts
Morning Zing Smoothie *Victoria Boutenko* 4:½ bunch dandelion greens 2 stalks celery ½ inch fresh gingerroot 2 peaches ½ pineapple Yields 2 quarts	**Party in Your Mouth** **Green Smoothie** *Sergei Boutenko* 1 small pineapple, cored 1 large mango, peeled ½ head romaine lettuce ½ inch fresh ginger root Yields 2 quarts
Rocket Fuel Smoothie *Victoria Boutenko* 2 cups green or red seedless grapes 3 golden kiwis, peeled 1 ripe orange, peeled, seeds removed 1 small leaf of aloe vera, with skin 5 leaves red leaf lettuce 2 cups water Yields 2 quarts	**Heavy Metals Be Gone** *Valya Boutenko* 1 bunch cilantro 2 cups stinging nettles 1 bunch fresh parsley 3 stalks celery 1 lemon, juiced 2 mangoes 2 cups apple juice Yields 2 quarts
Dark Green Love *Victoria Boutenko* 1 bunch dandelion greens 1 medium cucumber 3 cups water Yields 2 quarts	**Omega Aphrodisiac** *Victoria Boutenko* 3 cups wild purslane 1 small watermelon 3 limes, juiced Yields 2 quarts
Green Smoothie Monster *Victoria Boutenko* 4 leaves kale, stems removed 4 leaves chard, stems	**Summer Splendor** *Sergei Boutenko* 4 leaves chard, stems removed 3 stalks celery

removed	1 head fresh parsley
½ bunch fresh parsley	6 apricots
1 leaf aloe vera	3 peaches
½ bunch dandelion greens	½ vanilla bean
3 pears	Yields 2 quarts
1 banana	
3 cups water	
Yields 2 quarts	
"Bitter Delight" Cocktail *Victoria Boutenko*	**Revitalizing Energizer** *Victoria Boutenko*
1 large leaf aloe vera, with skin	6 young grape leaves (they contain resveratrol, which triggers longevity genes)
4 leaves chard, stems removed	3 leaves dinosaur kale, stems removed
3 cups chickweed	2 mangoes
1 banana	1 pint strawberries
1 peach	2 cups orange juice
1 pear	Yields 1 quart
Yields 1 quart	

c. 15 Green Smoothies in 3 Minutes - Video

Sergei Boutenko is in a video doing 15 green smoothies in 3 minutes - it was good.

#1. 1 Banana, 1 Papaya, 2 leaves Swiss Chard, 2 cups water

#2. 1 bunch Dandelions, 1 Banana, 1 Pear, 1 Mango, 2 cups water

#3. 3 leaves of Romaine Lettuce, ½ an Avocado, ½ Fuji Apple, 1 Banana, 2 cups water

#4. 5 leaves Purple Kale, ½ Orange, ½ Fuji Apple, small piece of Ginger, ½ an Avocado, Orange slices to decorate.

#5. 1 cup frozen Strawberries, 1 Banana, 1 Mango, 2 cups water, 2 leaves Rainbow Chard

#6. 1 large handful of Spinach, 1 Banana, 1 cup frozen Strawberries, 1 Orange, small piece of Ginger, 2 cups water

#7. 1 young Coconut, ½ of a small Pineapple, ½ Pear, 5 Leaves of Romaine Lettuce

#8. 1 cup frozen Raspberries, 5 leaves Red Leaf Lettuce, 1 Red Apple, 1 Green Apple, ½ of a small Pineapple, 2 cups water

#9. 1 large handful of Spinach, ¾ of Orange Bell Pepper, ½ an Avocado, 3 cloves Garlic, 2 Tomatoes, 2 cups of water (Savory Smoothie)

#10. ½ an Avocado, 2 Tomatoes, pinch of Cayenne Pepper, pinch of Salt, ½ of a Red Onion, 1 bunch Parsley, 1 Orange Bell Pepper, 2 cups water (Savory Smoothie)

#11. 2 Bananas, 3 pieces of Celery, 1 head of Red Leaf Lettuce, 2 cups water

#12. 2 leaves Purple Kale, 2 leaves Collard Greens, 2 Bananas, ½ an Asian Pear, 2 cups water, 1 cup frozen Raspberries

#13. 1 cup frozen Blueberries, ¼ pound Spinach, 1 Orange, 1 cup water

#14. 4 Tomatoes, 1 Red Bell Pepper, 1bunch Basil, ½ an Avocado

#15. 1 young Coconut, carrot tops from young carrots, ½ an Avocado 1 banana, 2 cups water.

d. What are some of the top Smoothie Ingredients people like?

This section was taken from a web blog "Renegade Health" asking about smoothie ingredients.[216] The first three letters of the name are mentioned and the dates of submission were between 3/26-28/2010. This gives a good review of different people in different parts of the country and what they like to add for a smoothie. It shows the variation and similarities in smoothie making. And it shows some of the excitement and enthusiasm in making smoothies.

The reason for this is to show the diversity and to show what is coming off the internet. It gives a basic feel as to what the smoothie community is about.

There's loads of things I like to put in green smoothies but my favorite, although I know some people don't approve, is virgin coconut oil. I really notice the difference in how I feel, if I leave it out so I just put in a spoonful along with whatever else I'm having. (Kir. 3/26-28/10)

Young coconut, the water and the meat. Goji berries, cacao and hemp seeds and whatever else I feel like adding that morning. Yummy! (Kay. 3/26-28/10)

Kale, romaine, tree collard leaf, parsley, 1 or 2 fruits (apple, banana, kiwi, pineapple, berries, etc.), spirolina, Vitamineral Green (a powder). (Bar. 3/26-28/10)

Oh wow – how can we pick just one? There are so many – I would have to say either hemp or chia seeds because I always include these in pretty much every smoothie. (Kat. 3/26-28/10)

Goji Berries! Spinach, Coconut, and … dulse. Yummy yummy. (Ter. 3/26-28/10)

I like to use a mango, strawberries, a little honey, Ormus Greens, spring lettuce, couple leaves of Kale, chia seeds and a little maca. Sometimes I'll add a pear or apple too if it's not sweet enough. (Mar. 3/26-28/10)

Kale, by far my favorite… with bananas, berries, peaches in the summer… yummmmm. (Chr. 3/26-28/10)

Kale, pineapple have been "showing up" a lot these days and chia seeds! (Zeb. 3/26-28/10)

This week my favorite is goji berries! It comes naturally to me to rotate my food, and in the process I usually obsess over one ingredient for a while. Was never into goji berries until this week. Probably my body's way of getting certain nutrients. (Ver. 3/26-28/10)

LOTS of greens, 1 apple, 1 whole lemon, fresh ginger, maybe a beet or carrot. Whatever I've got in the fridge. Made with a juicer (no pulp for me!) LOVE IT! I make enough for 2 servings and put the second one in a brown glass jar in the fridge for later. (Gia. 3/26-28/10)

My newest creation that I threw in the blender….a leftover salad of Alfalfa sprouts, spinach, Arugula and romaine with Banana, apple, orange, and fresh ginger. (Jo. 3/26-28/10)

SWISS CHARD … I have it growing in my front yard. awesome, organic, super easy… I use about 3 HUGE leaves (spine and all, of course! silly people who don't use the spine….) and add frozen organic berries, lemon, a banana with a LOT of cayenne and cinnamon. Oh and a tbsp of flax seed… (Mon. 3/26-28/10)

I make a "chewy" instead of a smoothie–I pulse the VitaMix instead of a full blend. First tons of greens: kale chard dandelion collards spinach, but just to bite size in water and ice. Then set that aside and in water and ice do cilantro or parsley with carrot burdock horseradish flax meal cucumber and lemon, pulsed to diced size. Add that to the greens. Then one large tomato fully blended. Shake it all up and eat it with a fork. I used to do fruit but it got too sweet and I guess greens taste good to me now. (Eli. 3/26-28/10)

Spinach, romaine, apple or banana, berries, bee pollen, goji berries, sometimes maca, some sort of green powder, dulse, and love! (3/26-28/10)

Normally in a smoothing I put cucumber, kale or spinach, coconut, raw honey (my favorite is wildflower honey) mango, pineapple, and whatever fruits are in season. (Bri. 3/26-28/10)

Just made a smoothie. Here's what I put in it. Banana, strawberries, water and a little almond milk, cinnamon, hemp seeds, chia seeds, lots of romaine lettuce and cilantro. YUM!! (Tyr. 3/26-28/10)

My favorite lately has been papaya, spinach, ginger, chia, coconut water and almond milk – so creamy and spicy with the ginger! Love it! (Lea. 3/26-28/10)

Great Topic! I have a lot of favorites. Depending on the season, pears, tangy apples, grapes, goji berries, mixed berries, oranges. Romaine lettuce, kale, baby spinach, mustard greens (when I'm brave), barley powder, ormus greens (give quite a kick). (Den. 3/26-28/10)

Kale, Parsley, Banana, Honey, Cinnamon, ginger root, Papaya, fresh lemon juice. I usually try for 3 fruits and 3 greens. Does not always happen. My smoothies vary with what is on sale or with the season! (Jan. 3/26-28/10)

e. Several Raw Chefs Smoothies

This sections is from various raw food chefs books on Smoothies and Raw Soups.

Julie Wandling in her book; *Thank God for Raw Recipes for Health*,[217] has a very simplified orientation on smoothies.

Blend the following ingredients in a blender to make some terrific treats:
1. **Carob**: frozen bananas, carob powered and vanilla rice or soy milk.
2. **Vanilla**: frozen bananas, vanilla soy or rice milk.
3. **Orange**: peeled/seeded oranges, ice cubes, frozen banana.
    (Sometimes we add coconut milk or dried coconut.)
4. **Berry**: frozen bananas, frozen berries (strawberry, raspberry, blueberry, blackberry:
    I pick and freeze tons of them when in season), vanilla soy or rice milk.
5. **Tropical**: frozen bananas, fresh or frozen mangos, pineapple, vanilla rice, soy milk, or coconut milk.

Several of Shazzi's Smoothies (Sharon Holdstock) from her book; *Shazzie's Detox Delights*.[218]	**Red and raw** 20 cherries, stoned 1 papaya, skinned and de-seeded 2 dates, stoned 10 strawberries
Green cream 1 cup of sprouted sunflower seeds 1 banana, peeled 2 kiwis, peeled Juice of 4 apples Blend all ingredients and drink	**Purple power** *This is my favorite drink in the world* 2 dates, stoned 4 bananas, peeled 1 punnet of blackberries ½ a pint of water Chop the dates. Blend all ingredients, strain and drink.

Matthew Kenney in his book; *Everyday Raw*,[219] has some unique smoothies.	**Immunity** 1 ½ cups frozen banana 1 packet (100g) frozen Acai 1 cup frozen blueberries 2 cups coconut water 1 teaspoon vanilla 1 pinch sea salt
The Blue Green 2 cups young coconut meat 2 teaspoons extra virgin coconut oil 4 teaspoons blue green algae ¼ cup agave 12 leaves fresh mint 3 cups coconut water 1 teaspoon vanilla 1 pinch sea salt Blend all ingredients	**Mint Cacao Cooler** ½ cup young coconut meat ½ cup agave ½ vanilla bean, scraped ¼ cup cacao nibs or cacao powder 2 cups Almond Milk 10 fresh mint leaves

There are some unique smoothies, drinks from Jeremy Safron and Renee Underkoffler in their book, *The Raw Truth the Art of Loving Foods.*[220]	**Fire Water** Serves 1-2 ½ gallon water 3 chili peppers sliced 1 lemon diced Juice of 1 orange 2 tsp beet powder Mix and serve
Green Dream Serves 1-2 2 ripe papayas 4 dates 1 cup coconut milk 4 frozen bananas 1-2 tbs. spirulina Pit dates and cover with	**Flaxative** Serves 1-2 ¼ cup flax seeds 1 ½ cup apple juice 2 frozen bananas Soak flax seed for 15 minutes. Drain. Blend flax and apple juice until smooth.

filtered water for 1 hour. Blend dates and soak water until smooth. Blend date mixture, papayas and coconut milk. Blend in frozen bananas and spirulina.	Blend in bananas until smooth.

Nomi Shannon in her book, *The Raw Gourmet*,[221] gives some interesting smoothies.	**Milk and Fruit Smoothie** 1 cup grain milk or nut or seed milk 1 frozen banana, cut in chunks 2 frozen strawberries Blend until smooth.
Carob Shake 3-4 dates, pitted, soaked for 20 minutes 1 cup nut or grain milk 1 frozen banana, cut in chunks 3-4 tablespoons carob powder Dash vanilla (optional) Soak dates for 20 minutes and blend.	**Frozen Vanilla Bliss** ¾ cup water 2 tablespoons raw tahini, or more to taste 1-2 frozen bananas, cut in chunks Dash vanilla (optional) Blend until thick and smooth.

Alissa Cohen, in her book, *Living on Live Food*,[222] gives some simple but great smoothies.	**Green Apple and Parsley** 4 green apples ½ head parsley Juice all ingredients through a juicer
Mudslide ½ cup almonds 1 ½ cups water 1 banana	**Chocolate Mocha Milkshake** ½ cup sesame seeds 2 cups coconut milk

3 dates Blend until smooth.	½ cup coconut meat 1 Tablespoon honey 1 tbsp carob powder 1 banana In a blender, blend until smooth.

B. Smoothie Puddings

Some of the smoothies can be used as a pudding by leaving out the water or other liquids so that it remains thick. So it becomes a choice blend them with more liquid and it becomes a smoothie, blend with less liquid and it becomes a pudding.

Smoothie Puddings from Jim Tibbetts	
Avoca-Berry-Carrot Jim Tibbetts 1 avocado ¼ cup carrot juice ¼ cup berry juice 1 scoop protein powder	**Avoca-Kiwi-Orange** Jim Tibbetts 1 kiwi ½ avocado 2 tbsp almond butter 1 small orange 1 cup banana strawberry smoothie from store
Avoca-Mango-Cuke Jim Tibbetts ½ avocado 2 tbsp almond butter ¼ cup carrot juice ¼ cup mango juice ¼ cup cucumber juice 1 scoop protein powder	**Cucumber High** Jim Tibbetts ¼ cup carrot juice ¼ cup cucumber juice 1 cup green fruit juice smoothie from store 1 cucumber 1 bunch baby spinach 2 tbsp almond butter 1 scoop protein powder

Down to Earth Smoothie	Tomato Mango Twist
Jim Tibbetts	Jim Tibbetts
1 avocado	1 tomato
1 cucumber	½ avocado
1 cup baby spinach	1 cup baby spinach
1 cup strawberry banana	2 cups mango smoothie
fruit juice smoothie	1 cup water
1 tbsp almond butter	1 tbsp almond butter
1 scoop protein powder	1 scoop protein powder
Honeydew Berry Veggie	**Blue-Red and Yellow**
Jim Tibbetts	Jim Tibbetts
1 banana	1 cucumber
1 avocado	1 tomato
½ honeydew melon	1 cup baby spinach
1 cup berry veggie juice	1 slice pineapple
from	½ cup coconut yogurt
the store	½ cup blueberries
2 tbsp protein powder	1 scoop protein powder

Puddings from Victoria and Valya	
Kent Mango Bliss	**Green Pudding**
Victoria Boutenko	*Victoria Boutenko*
2 Kent mangoes	1 bunch fresh parsley
1 bunch chard, stems	5 grape leaves
removed	½ pineapple
1 pear	1 Abbot pear
1 banana	1 orange, peeled
Serve with kiwi.	1 cup water
Yields 3 cups	Yields 2 cups
Persimmon Pudding	**Applesauce Pudding**
Victoria Boutenko	*Valya Boutenko*
3 fuyu persimmons, peeled,	4 apples
seeds removed	1 banana
3 cups baby spinach	1 head romaine lettuce
1 ripe banana	½ teaspoon cinnamon
Yields 2 cups	2 cups water
	Yields 3 cups

C. Smoothie Soups

a. Warming and Raw Soups

Raw soups are soups that are not cooked and most books on raw receipts have different soups that are raw. Warming soups have heat added to them. Living Food Soups do not include grain based pasta, which is a dead food.

Warm soups can be made by a person into raw foods and living foods but they cannot be cooked soups. To make this distinction we call them "Warming soups" because they are warming to the inside and to the taste. In order to do this it means using two pans to prepare the soups. In the first pan goes all the veggies and some or all of the liquids or foods that are only to be warmed and not cooked. In the second pan goes all the foods that are to be cooked, meaning brought to a boil. Whenever something is boiled or cooked most of the nutrient value is lost.

Never boil vegetables, at boiling the vegetables will be almost destroyed in nutrient value. All water soluble vitamins are destroyed over 150 degrees, at boiling 212 degrees the nutritional value is greatly destroyed, even proteins start to become denatured. Anything over 120 degrees destroys the enzymes.

Warming Soups are hot but the warming pan never reaches boiling or if it does it is turned off to cook, it is only slightly warmed. The cooked pan can be boiled to prepare that section of the food. Then the foods in the cooked pan are added to the warmed pan, and the soup is done!

There are three ways to do Warming Soups: chunky, creamed or both together. For chunky soups just cup the veggies up into small chunks. For creamed soups put the produce and other foods like nuts into a blender or food

116

processor like a Cuisinart and blend it down into a cream base and add it to the soup. Or you can make part of it chunky and part of it a cream base and add them together.

Scuba Diving Soup Jim Tibbetts	Space Walk Soup Jim Tibbetts
Warming soup part 4 carrots cut into pieces ½ cabbage cut into slices 1 eggplant cut into cubes ¼ cup sunflower seeds ¼ cup pumpkin seeds 2 tbsp miso 1 sweet potato blended ½ orange pepper blended ½ broccoli blended ¼ fennel blended 2 cups water Cooked soup part 2 cups water 2 small onions Several garlic pieces Spices to taste	Warming soup part 2 cup water ¼ cup broccoli ¼ cup lettuce ¼ cup carrot ¼ cup fennel ¼ cup parsley 1 small piece green onion Veggies dice into pieces, blending optional 1 cup squash – blended 1 tbsp miso soup mix 1 tbsp flax oil 1 tbsp apple cider vinegar Cooked soup part 1 slice onion 1 piece garlic Dash salt, Dash rosemary, Dash cilantro
Tomato-Veggie-Broccoli Jim Tibbetts	Broccoli Carrot Soup Jim Tibbetts

Warming soup part
Organic Crushed tomatoes
    w/basil (can)
1 cup broccoli diced
½ cup hard veggies Salad
(beets, celery, green
squash, yellow squash,
cauliflower, turnips, orange
pepper.
	Warming soup part
	Organic Crushed tomatoes
	    w/basil (can)
	2 whole tomatoes cut up
	1 cup celery diced
	½ cup hard veggies Salad
	(beets, celery, green squash,
	yellow squash, cauliflower,
	turnips, orange pepper.

117

Cooked soup part 1 red onion diced ½ cup cooked separately sweet potato diced Spices: Thyme leaves, kelp granules, dulse granules, 2 tbsp lemon juice.	Cooked soup part ½ cup cooked separately sweet potato diced ¼ red onion diced 8 small green onions diced Spices: Thyme leaves, kelp granules, dulse granules, 2 tbsp lemon juice.

Sweet Potato-Veggie Soup
Jim Tibbetts
 	
Warming soup part
1 cup water
3 small carrots
1 stick celery
Slice red cabbage
¼ yellow pepper
Slice onion
1 clove garlic
1 cup pate (sweet potato,
soaked almonds ground,
blended into a pate)
Spices
Kelp granules
Seasoning (oregano, basil,
marjoram, garlic)
 	
Cooked soup part
1 red onion diced
½ cup cooked separately
sweet potato diced
Spices: Thyme leaves, kelp
granules, dulse granules.
	Tomato-Veggie-Yams
	Jim Tibbetts
	
	Warming soup part
	Organic Crushed tomatoes
	  w/basil (can)
	2 whole tomatoes cut up
	1 cup celery diced
	½ cup hard veggies Salad
	(beets, celery, green squash,
	yellow squash, cauliflower,
	turnips, orange pepper.
	
	Cooked soup part
	½ cup cooked separately
	sweet
	   potato diced
	¼ red onion diced
	8 small green onions diced
	Spices: Thyme leaves, kelp
	granules, dulse granules,
	2 tbsp lemon juice.

Squash Soup; Turnip Soup, Possible Variations
Jim Tibbetts

Main Broth
1 or 2 Squash
1 or 2 Turnip

Veggie - 1 to 3
Onions
Garlic
Red or green Peppers
Beets

Nuts and Seeds - 1 or 2
Walnuts
Pine Nuts
Sunflower seeds
Pistachio

Liquids
Water
Coconut juice
Fruit Juice
Vegetable Juice

Seasonings - 1 to 3
Pepper
Salt
Oregano
Sage
Yellow Mustard seed
All Seasoning

Optional
1 T. Protein powder
1 T. Olive Oil
    or flax or hemp
1 T. Honey or Maple syrup

Example "mmm" Soup
1 large squash
1/8 small onion
1/8 orange pepper
1 clove garlic

1/8 cup walnuts
1/8 cup pine nuts

dash black pepper
dash yellow mustard seed
dash herbal seasoning

1 teaspoon protein powder
1 teaspoon flax oil
1 teaspoon maple syrup

One large or two small squash are needed. Cut in squares and heat the squash up till it is warm. Put it in the Cusinart and blend it up to a sauce. Soak the nuts and seeds for 10 to 25 minutes then drain off the liquid. Add a little water, some seasonings, then the veggies and nuts into the squash broth and mix it up, heating if necessary but do not boil.

Optional
add some protein powder, sweetener and/or oil.

Season to taste	Of course change the veggies, nuts and seeds as suits your taste.

b. Selected Raw Chefs Soups

At the Hippocrates Health Institute several green soups are given by Anna Maria Clement, and Kelly Serbonich in their book, *Healthful Cuisine.*[223]

Hippocrates' Green Soup Anna Maria Clement, and Kelly Serbonich	**Kelly's Favorite Super Green Soup** Kelly Serbonich
Yield: 4 cups 1-1 ¾ cups chopped fresh herbs of your choice 1 cup chopped cucumber ½ avocado ½ cup chopped celery ¼ cup chopped scallion ¾ teaspoon kelp powder 2 cups green juice* 1 teaspoon fresh lemon juice, optional Combine all ingredients, blend well and season to taste.	Yield: 2 ½ cups 2 cups chopped dark leafy greens ½ cup whole leaf dulse, snipped into pieces ¼ cup chopped scallion ¼ cup sauerkraut 1 cup water or green juice* (below) In a blender, combine all ingredients. Blend well and season to taste. Serve.
*Hippocrates' Green Juice: Yield 2 cups 1 ½ cucumbers, 3 stalks of celery, 4 cups combination of sunflower and pea green sprouts. Feed ingredients through a single or double auger juicer. Drink within	**Spinach Mint Soup** Yield: 2-4 servings 1 cup fresh cucumber juice 1 cup chopped spinach 1/3 cup chopped red onion 1/3 cup chopped red bell pepper ¼ cup chopped fresh mint

20 minutes for optimal nutrition. Other greens that are commonly used to make green juice: kale, Swiss chard, parsley, spinach, lettuce and beet. In a blender, combine all ingredients. Blend well and season to taste. Serve.	¼ avocado 1 clove garlic 2 cups water 2 tbsp Bragg Liquid Aminos or Nama Shoyu In a blender, combine all ingredients. Blend until smooth and season to taste. Serve.

Rhio has some great soups in her book: *Hooked on Raw,* *Rejuvenate Your Body and* *Soul with Nature's Living* *Foods*[224]	**Borscht** 1 medium beet 5 large carrots 1 lemon, peeled ½ large cucumber minced 1-2 shallots, minced 1 scallion, minced 2 heaping tbsp. red lentil sprouts (optional) 2 heaping tbsp. any non-dairy yogurt or plain seed cheese 1) In a juicer, prepare beet, carrot and lemon juices. 2) Top each bowl with rest of the ingredients

Almond Creamy Soup
  (Base for 100 soups)
1 ½ cups sprouted almonds, blanched
2 cups filtered water
2 lemons, juiced
1 garlic clove
1 tbsp. flaxseed oil
½ tsp. ground cumin
½ tsp. Celtic sea salt
1 tsp Vegetable Seasoning
   and Broth
	Green Powder Soup
	
	2 cups cucumber juice
	2 ½ cups of Greens (kale, chard, beet tops or others)*
	¼ - ½ avocado
	¼ - ½ lemon, juiced
	1 garlic clove
	1-2 tsp. mellow white miso (optional)
	1) Prepare the cucumber juice in a juicer, (or other

Dash of Nama Shoyu
  (optional)
Put all ingredients into a
blender, this is the base.
Add in the following or
make your own add in:

Lemon Zucchini Bisque:
2 small zucchini, grated
½ cup finely minced shallot
(or onion)

Corn-Off-The-Cob:
1 corn, cut off the cob
¼ cup minced shallot
¼ red bell pepper, chopped
2 mushrooms, chopped

Almond-Beet Borscht
½ beet, grated
½ cup chopped cucumber
¼ cup finely minced chives
or chopped dill.

green juice) then put it into
a blender with all the rest of
the ingredients and blend to
a creamy consistency.
2) Any sprouts which you
have on hand such as lentils,
wild rice, mung beans, etc.
can be spooned on top of
the soup before serving.

*The greens can be
marinated because most
people are not accustomed
yet to the raw taste.

	Cream of Carrot Soup
	3 carrots, chopped
Gabriel Cousens, MD	2 stalks of celery
Has some chefs at his	2 C almonds, soaked
Tree of Life Rejuvenation	2-3 cloves of garlic
Center give receipts	2 C water
in his book:	1 ½ C orange juice
Rainbow Green Live-Food	1 t nutmeg
Cuisine[225]	In a blender, process all ingredients until smooth and creamy.
Fennel Soup	**Green Campfire Stew**
2 C Fennel bulb, chopped	
1 C tomato	2 C avocado
1 ½ T lemon juice	2 C water
½ T garlic, minced	1 C fresh cilantro,
½ t oregano	de-stemmed and minced
½ t sage	1 C celery
1/2 t Celtic salt	½ C kale, de-stemmed
½ C avocado, diced	½ C lemon or lime juice
½ C cucumber, diced	2 T Celtic salt
1/3 C red bell pepper,	1 t cayenne pepper
diced	1 hot pepper, seeded
In a blender, process fennel, tomato, lemon juice, garlic, oregano, sage, and Celtic salt until smooth and liquefied. Strain the mixture and stir in avocado, cucumber, and red bell peppers. Garnish with fresh herbs. Serves 2-3.	Combine all ingredients in blender and mix until thoroughly creamy. Serve immediately.

Victoria, Valya, Sergei Boutenko Soups	
Cucumber Dill-icious Soup *Valya Boutenko* 2 cucumbers ½ bunch dill 1 large avocado 5 leaves dinosaur kale, stems removed 2 stalks celery 1 lime, juiced 3 cloves garlic Yields 2 quarts	**Mediterranean Soup** *Victoria Boutenko* 3 cups spinach 3 stalks celery 1 sprig oregano 1 sprig thyme 1 red bell pepper 1 large avocado 1 cucumber 1 jalapeño pepper 1 lime, juiced 2 cups water Enjoy with dulse leaves or flakes. Yields 3 quarts
Soup Gazpacho *Victoria Boutenko* 3 leaves kale, stems removed 1 bunch basil 3 large tomatoes 2 stalks celery 1 red bell pepper 1 large avocado 1 lime, juiced 1 cup water 2 cups love Yields 2 quarts	**Thai Soup** *Sergei Boutenko* 2 cucumbers 1 large avocado 1 lime, juiced 3 cloves garlic 6 leaves curly kale, stems removed ½ teaspoon dried turmeric powder ½ inch fresh gingerroot 2 cups water Yields 2 quarts

D. Salads and Salad Soups

There are thousands of ways to make salads and there are many books out with many great salads. In this book it is only teaching you how to make two salads. One is the "Hard Salads" and the other is the "Soft Salads". Then I will show you how to take one or both of these and use them in a soup.

When talking about salads and salad soups I am talking about fruits, vegetables, nuts, seeds, sprouted legumes and sprouted grains. We are not talking about grain based flours turned into pasta or legumes/grains/beans that are cooked down to a mush. These are dead or dormant foods and all soups and salads and smoothies need to be or are best as Living Foods! Pasta and most processed foods have little to no nutritional value and may be counterproductive to ones' health.

The whole point of this lifestyle is the focus on Living Foods and not dead or dormant foods; this is a diet, a nutritional program that is based on the Culture of Life and not the Culture of Death and degenerative disease.

Hard Veggie Salad
First is the standard hard vegetable salad, which is just what it says it is made up of the hard vegetables that you grow or buy in the store. Take as many as you want of these hard veggies and put them through a food processor like a Cusinart. This would slice them up to a small size. Of the 14 hard vegetables listed below at times we have used all 14 for one salad! But most of the time it is between 6 to 12 different hard vegetables that are put through a food processor for the salad. But in making a salad this way it is easy to make more than one salad at a time.

Standard Hard Veggie Salad	
Celery	Asparagus
Carrots	Red Cabbage
Broccoli	Cauliflower
Yellow Squash	Green beans
Zucchini	Yellow pepper
Beets	Orange pepper
Turnips	Other hard veggies
Green onions (scallions)	Other combinations

By making more than one salad this way several salads can be made. Usually we would take and spend an hour or two making a big batch of hard vegetable salads putting them in containers, enough for a whole week. Some of them can be put in smaller containers that can be taken to work. These hard vegetables cut up will easily last for a week in the refrigerator.

The "Soft Salads" are all the softer vegetables such as cucumber, tomatoes, spinach and other softer vegetables that might be used. The soft vegetables if cut up in a food processor do not always last a week. In-addition they are also watery and could start to soften the hard vegetables which could make them go bad quicker. So while making up the Hard Veggies you can also make up the Soft Veggies but put them in a separate container. These Soft Veggies can be put in with the Hard Veggies when you are to have a salad or they can be served as a vegetable dish on their own. Sometime we have a big bowl of hard veggies with a salad dressing and a smaller bowl of soft veggies in oil.

Soup-Hard Veggie Salad Combo
A Soup-Salad Combo is simply a soup base with hard vegetables (or some soft vegetables) added to it. Such as take a can of tomato puree or diced or chunks as the soup base heat it up, add spices or onions and/or garlic to make the base. This can be cooked to taste. Then when that is ready take it off the burner and start to let it cool. Then add the

Hard Veggie salad such as: cauliflower, cabbage, turnips, parsnips, carrots, beets, and asparagus.

Soup Base with Spices added
- Can of tomato puree or diced or chunks
- Sweet Potatoes
- Miso soup base
- Other soup base

Soup Hard Veggies
Cauliflower, cabbage, turnips, parsnips, carrots, beets, asparagus, etc.

Any combination of Hard Veggies can be used, or Soft Veggies can be used this is your choice. The spices are best to be cooked and the soup base is usually cooked and the spices can be added to it. The vegetables themselves should not be cooked but only heated up or added to a hot soup base. Some of the vegetables like onions or garlic may need to be cooked in the soup base or separately and added to the soup.

Cooking and boiling vegetables is not needed, yet some vegetables that might disagree with a person when eaten raw; such as onions and garlic, can be cooked. Any combination of spices can be added to the cooked soup base.

To add some heat in terms of spice to a salad or pate a small side dish as a Hot Salad Add-in could be added to salads, soups, pates or even smoothies.

Hot Salad Add-in	
1 red pepper	6 small radishes
1 yellow pepper	1 carrot
1 small green jalapeno pepper	2 small red jalapeno peppers
1 Tbsp Miso	Ginger dressing
1 small onion	¼ teaspoon turmeric
½ garlic, all cloves	¼ teaspoon curry power

E. Pates and Paté Short Soups

A Paté is using a sweet potato or a small pumpkin, or a small squash or other similar vegetable to put into a blender and blend it, and add various ingredients to it. The Paté can be eaten like potatoes or they can have vegetables added or extra liquid added to make a Paté soup. Short Soups means "short of cooking" since they are warmed up.

These "Paté Short Soups" are really pate's with salad material added then some spices are added to and put in hot water, but never boiling water. The term "Short" is to indicate a short or small heating time. Always the spices are put in first and simmered only for a minute or two. Then some hard or harsh vegetables are put in that may be easier to eat if simmered for a minute or two, such as garlic, onion, broccoli, hot peppers, etc. These also are never boiled just warmed up for a minute or two. Then finally the rest of the vegetables are put in and only for a minute are they left on the stove and then the heat is turned off.

Never boil vegetables, at boiling the vegetables will be destroyed in nutrient value. All water soluble vitamins are destroyed over 150 degrees, at boiling 212 degrees the nutritional value is greatly destroyed, even proteins start to become denatured. Anything over 120 degrees destroys the enzymes. That is why the vegetables are always thrown in last, and then never left in for more than a minute or two. The temperature is one factor and the time element is the second factor in cooking. If you simmer something for 5-10 minutes it is like boiling it for 1-2 minutes. Cooking is usually associated with longer lengths of time. That is why this approach is really warming soups and not cooking the foods.

These veggie short soups are really salads (without dressing) that some spices are added to and put in hot water, but never boiling water. Always the spices are put in first and simmered only for a minute or two since they often taste better that way. Then some hard or spicy vegetables are put in that may be easier to eat if simmered for a minute or two, such as garlic, onion, broccoli, hot peppers, etc. Some people have a hard time with some types of raw vegetables like onion or garlic. These also are never boiled just warmed up for a minute or two. Then finally the rest of the vegetables are put in and only for a minute are they left on the stove and then the heat is turned off. This approach allows the spices to simmer and give off their flavor yet it is only to heat the foods up for a minute or two and not to cook it. Boiling only ends up weakening and destroying the nutritional value of the food. Remember we want Live Foods!

Straightforward Paté Jim Tibbetts	Simple Garlic Paté Jim Tibbetts
1 sweet potato ¼ cup almonds soaked ¼ cup leeks Parsley as garnish Sea salt to taste	1 sweet potato Handful almonds soaked 1 clove garlic 1 tbsp organic lemon juice 1 tbsp flax seed oil 1 tbsp E3 Live Dash oregano Dash sea salt
Red Pumpkin Short Soup Jim Tibbetts	**Spiced Sweet Potato Short Soup** Jim Tibbetts
1 – cup water ½ - small pumpkin 1 – clove garlic Handful – baby spinach Slices – red cabbage Spices: Kelp granules, oregano, caraway seeds	Simmer Spices: for a minute or two: salt, kelp, savory Add: 1 – sweet potato Slice – onions Slice – garlic 1 tbsp – flaxseed oil Have the soup cold, room

Have the soup cold, room temperature or
    Simmer for a minute and turn off.
	temperature or
	    Simmer for a minute and turn off.

Cabbage Kale Short Soup
Jim Tibbetts
 	
Bring to a simmer 1 cup water:
    Add <u>Spices:</u>
Marjoram, savory, celery salt
    Simmer one minute and add:
Slices – red cabbage
Handful – kale
1 – sweet potato
1 – slice garlic
1 – small tomato
   Have the soup cold, room temperature or
    Simmer one minute and turn off.
	Squash-star Short Soup
	Jim Tibbetts
	
	Simmer 1 cup water with:
	    <u>Spices:</u>
	Kelp granules, salt, oregano
	    <u>Add:</u>
	1 – small squash
	1 – garlic clove
	Slice – onion
	1 tbsp – oil
	1 tbsp – honey
	   Have the soup cold, room temperature or
	    Simmer one minute and turn off.

Superman Paté Soup
Jim Tibbetts
 	
Simmer two cups water:
Rosemary, Savory,
Crushed Mint
Onions, Garlic
 	
    <u>Blend Paté:</u>
Sweet potato
Parsley
Fennel
 	
    <u>Add:</u> the Blended Paté to soup. Have the soup
	Racecar Paté Soup
	Jim Tibbetts
	
	½ small pumpkin
	1 – sweet potato
	1 – clove garlic
	Slice – cabbage
	Bunch - baby spinach
	
	    <u>Spices:</u>
	Dash – celery salt
	Dash – crushed mint
	   Have the soup cold, room temperature or
	    Simmer for a minute and

cold, room temperature or simmer for a minute and turn off.	turn off.

Skydiving Paté Soup
    Jim Tibbetts
 	
1 – Sweet potato
1 – clove garlic
¼ - onion
¼ cup – almonds (soaked, blended)
    Spices:
Caraway seeds, savory, kelp granules
  Have the soup cold, room temperature or
    Simmer for a minute and turn off.
	Over the Hill Paté
	    Jim Tibbetts
	
	    Blend Paté:
	1 – sweet potato
	½ - lemon
	1 – green onion
	1 – slice onion
	    Herbs:
	Oregano, basil, marjoram, garlic.
	Have the soup cold, room temperature or
	    Simmer for a minute and turn off.

Beach bum Paté
    Jim Tibbetts
 	
1 – Sweet Potato
1 – Tomato
Several pieces broccoli
1 – clove garlic
Slice – onion
    Herbs:
Dash Himalayan salt
Dash cilantro
2 tbsp E-3 Live
Have the soup cold, room temperature or
    Simmer for a minute and turn off.
	Yellow Submarine Paté
	    Jim Tibbetts
	
	1 – sweet potato
	1 – clove garlic
	Slices – red cabbage
	Handful – baby spinach
	1 tbsp – honey
	
	Spices to taste.
	Have the soup cold, room temperature or
	    Simmer for a minute and turn off.

Green Dragon Paté
    Jim Tibbetts
 	
1 piece broccoli
1 piece yellow pepper
	Backstage Paté Soup
	    Jim Tibbetts
	
	Cut up 2 cups of mixed vegetables

1 piece green onion ½ avocado ½ yellow sweet potato ½ gold sweet potato 1 clove garlic 1 tbsp flax oil 1 tbsp E-3 live Dash kelp powder Dash marjoram herb Have the soup cold, room temperature or Simmer for a minute and turn off.	Carrot Red cabbage Celery Cilantro herbs 1 cup water ½ sweet potato 4 cups soaked almonds Bring one cup water to simmer with sweet potato and almonds and salt. Add the 2 cups of veggies to warm take off heat.
Lakeview Paté Soup Jim Tibbetts 1 ½ cup water ½ yellow squash ¼ cup almonds soaked ground 2 sticks carrots ¼ cup broccoli ¼ cup cauliflower 1 tbsp *E3 Live* 1 tbsp apple cider vinegar 1 tbsp *Odo's oil* 1 tbsp herbal mixture Dash oregano, Himalayan salt	**Fall Weather Paté Soup** Jim Tibbetts 1 cup water 1 sweet potato ¼ cup soaked almonds 1 handful cauliflower 2 stalks celery 1 small beet Herbs: Oregano, basil, marjoram, garlic, little salt
Kale Cabb Paté Soup Jim Tibbetts 1 cup water 1 sweet potato 1 handful kale 1 handful red cabbage ¼ orange pepper ½ handful cilantro Dash: Himalayan salt,	**Coconut Sweet Potato** Jim Tibbetts ½ cup almonds soaked ½ squash ½ sweet potato 1 tbsp Udo's 3-6-9 oil 1 tbsp Dulse Granules (seaweed) ½ tbsp miso (barley miso)

crushed mint, oregano.	¼ cup shredded coconut
Miso Sweet Potato Soup Jim Tibbetts ½ cup almonds soaked 1 sweet potato 1 tbsp Udo's 3-6-9 oil 1 tbsp Triple Blend Sea Flakes ½ tbsp miso (barley miso) ¼ cup shredded coconut	**Veggie Basic Soup** Jim Tibbetts 1 cup water ¼ cup broccoli ¼ cup lettuce ¼ cup carrot ¼ cup fennel ¼ cup parsley 1 small piece green onion Have the soup cold, or simmer for a minute.

Some of the soups and foods have a little heating or even cooking, this is to accommodate for the people who are in the state of transition. It takes time for most people to adapt to a raw vegan or a Living Foods lifestyle. Having a little of the foods cooked, warmed or heated helps in that transition and also it is comforting or comfort foods, for those not yet adapted to living raw foods.

To restate the reason behind this type of nutritional approach is that the whole point of this lifestyle is the focus on Living Foods and not dead foods, this is a nutritional program that is based on the Culture of Life and not the Culture of Death and degenerative disease. This dietary lifestyle is designed to bring health and healing to the person: body and soul.

IX. Spiritual Nutrition

Spiritual Nutrition implies that there is a spiritual connection and roots. Back in Biblical times everything was natural and organic, there was no mercury in the water or toxins in the air or factory farming. They had a great concern for purity of body and soul to such a degree that many ate a plant based diet, a kosher vegetarian diet. There is the belief that Jesus himself was a vegetarian. Let us look into this to give a spiritual foundation for the emphasis in this book.

A. Purification of the Body

In the Old Testament, it teaches us in the Jewish lineage that three times a day the Jews should recite the Shelma (Deut 6.5), which includes - love God with all your strength/body! We need knowledge so as not to destroy ourselves or sin. There is a way that is right and leads through a narrow gate but takes strength. Finally we must renew our minds and be transformed for what is the good and acceptable Will of God. In the beginning God gave us a plant-based lifestyle that shall be our food.

- "The Lord is our God, the Lord alone! Therefore, you shall love the Lord, your God, with all your heart, and with all your soul, and with all your strength (body)." Deut 6.5; Lk 10:25
- The prophet Hosea said to the kingdom of Judah, "My people are destroyed from lack of knowledge." Hosea 4:6
- The sin of omission is found in James: "To know good and not to do it for him it is a sin." James 4:17
- "There is a way that some think right, but it leads in the end to death." Pr 16.25
- "Strive to enter through the narrow gate, for many, I tell you, will attempt to enter but will not be strong enough." Luke 13:23
- And be not conformed to this world; but be ye transformed by the renewing of your mind, that ye

may prove what is that good and acceptable and perfect Will of God." Romans 12:2

- God's first dietary command: "God said, 'See, I give you all the seed-bearing plants that are upon the whole earth, and all the trees with seed-bearing fruit; this shall be your food." Gen 1:29

The act of eating food is for the sake of purification or detoxification. Junk Foods, Comfort Foods, Fast Foods are "Delicacies" or the "Kings Foods" in scripture. The sin of gluttony means eating too much food or too much of the wrong types of food.

- Avoiding certain foods is needed to avoid addictions. "Let not my heart be drawn to what is evil, to take part in wicked deeds with men who are evildoers; let me not eat of their delicacies." (Ps 141:4)
- "When you sit down to dine with a ruler, keep in mind who is before you; put a knife to your throat if you have a ravenous appetite. Do not desire his delicacies; they are deceitful food." Pr 23.1-3
- "My son, test your soul while you live; see what is bad for it and do not give it that. For not everything is good for everyone, and not every person enjoys everything. Do not have an insatiable appetite for any luxury, and do not give yourself up to food; for overeating brings sickness, and gluttony leads to nausea. Many have died of gluttony, but he who is careful to avoid it prolongs his life." Sirach 37:27-31

As St. Paul says, in 1 Corinthians and other texts that there is a strong emphasis on the wholeness and holiness of the body as noted in these verses:

- "Your body, you know, is the temple of the Holy Spirit, who is in you since you received him from God." (1 Cor 6:19) "If anybody should destroy the temple of God, God will destroy him, because the temple of God is sacred, and you are that temple." 1 Cor 3.17
- "Whatever you eat, whatever you drink, whatever you do at all, do it for the glory of God." 1 Cor 11.31

- "I have told you often, and I repeat it today with tears, there are many who are behaving as the enemies of the cross of Christ. They are destined to be lost. They make food into their god." (Phil 3:18, 19) "I have learned how to cope with every circumstance - how to eat well or go hungry, to be well provided for or do without." Phil 4:12
- "A man never hates his own body, but he feeds it and looks after it; and that is the way Christ treats the Church, because it is his body - and we are its living parts." Eph 5:29
- "May the God of peace make you perfect and holy. May He preserve you whole and entire, spirit, soul and body, irreproachable for the coming of our Lord Jesus Christ." 1 Thess 5.23

B. Fasting and Healing

Fasting is a main means of detoxification or purification. If Moses, who beheld God, (on Sinai) and St. Paul, the divine apostle (Act 9:9) fasted, so must we. If the Ninevites fasted (Jonah 3:5), and this included all their children plus their 'senior' citizens, so we must. If the Church Fathers and the Saints fasted, and expected others to fast, so must we. Finally, if Jesus Himself fasted and was hungry (Lk 4:2), who are we to introduce a 'new improved and fast-free' spirituality?'

Fasting is found throughout the Bible and was a major part of the faith and practice.
- "He (Jesus) fasted for forty days and forty nights, after which he was very hungry." Mt 4:2
  Afterwards, "Jesus, returned in the power of the Spirit to Galilee." Lk 4:14
- Jesus gave an admonition telling people: "Moreover, when you fast..." Mt 6:16
- And at the death of Saul, "they fasted for seven days." 1 Ch 10:12, 1 Sam 31:13.
- "But now, now - it is Yahweh who speaks - come back to me with all your heart, fasting, weeping,

mourning." Joel 2:12

- "Repentance to conquer addictions is needed: 'We afflict our souls (Lev 23:27, 32) by fasting (cf. Ezra 8:21) and repenting of one's sins (Ezek 18:30-31)." 'Repent, and turn from all your transgressions, so that iniquity will not be your ruin.'" Ezek 18:20-21

In Biblical times for a person to be cured meant that they were purified or cleansed. Purify is mentioned as one of the means of the four definitions of healing. Healing indeed plays a large role in the Gospel, where four different verbs are used to express it.

- One is *therepeuo*, which is used forty-two times in the New Testament (Mt 16; Mk 6; Lk 13; Jn 1; Ac 4; Apoc 2)
- Another is *iaomai* (*iatros*, 'physician,' is a noun from the same root), which is used twenty-six times in the New Testament, especially by Luke, who was himself a physician (Lk 11; Ac 4; Mt 4; scattered use in other New Testament books.)
- A third is *katharizo*, which means "purify" (Mt 8:2,3; 11:5; Mk 1:40; Lk 5:12; 17:14), (used many times in Old Testament).
- The fourth verb is *sozein*, "save," which is often used of "salvation" in the full and transcendent sense, but is also used in the sense of "heal" (notably in Mt 9:21-22; 14:36; Mk 5:23, 28; 6:56; Lk 7:3; 8:36, 48 50; 17:19; Jn 11:12; Ac 4:9; 14:9; Jm 5:15).

C. Kosher, Pure Foods

Kosher means pure foods it is a basic principle in the Bible, first emphasized in Genesis then in the other books of the Bible. Rabbi Noach Valley points out that: "In the Torah it is written, 'You shall be holy because I, Adonai your God, am holy' (Leviticus 10:2). Every one of us Jews is commanded to be holy. Holiness, in Judaism, is in the nature of an 'imitation of God.' For example, holiness and not health or hygiene is the reason for the laws of kashrut."[226]

Richard Schwartz, Ph.D. is one of the leading writers of a vegetarian Judaism. (book: *Judaism and Vegetarianism)* points out: "There is no contradiction between Judaism (and its dietary laws) and vegetarianism. In fact, Jewish vegetarians argue that vegetarianism is the diet most consistent with the highest Jewish values."[227]

The early Jewish Scriptures and lifestyle emphasized kindness to animals: "And you shall walk in His ways." Deut 28.9 "Thou shall not kill." Ex 20.13 "His (Yahweh's) compassion is over all His creatures." Ps 145.9

The words "clean" or "unclean" and "purification" or "to be purified" occur over five hundred times in the Bible, it was a major concept and concern to Biblical writers. There is a close relationship between the terms, "uncleanness" and "sin." And it was usually the priests job to "separate the sacred from the profane, the unclean from the clean."[228] The term has numerous forms such as cleanness;[229] to cleanse; to cleanse oneself; purifying; cleansing; clean; in the purifying rituals 'to sin' is normally translated as 'to cleanse'[230], and to cleanse oneself; morally clean.[231] (cleanness (Lev 15:13; 22:4); to cleanse (Lev 16:30; Num 8:6); to cleanse oneself (Num 8:7; Josh 22:17); purifying (Lev 12:4); cleansing (Lev 13:7: Num 6:9); clean (Gen 7:2; Lev 11:47)

The unclean is prohibited or repulsive to God,[232] or it belongs to the realm of the demonic which is opposed to God, and uncleanness is described as an abomination to Yahweh. Since Yahweh was a moral God he demanded ethical purity "clean hands and a pure heart" (Ps 24:4). There is a close connection between holiness and cleanliness, but they are not the same. The Day of Atonement (a day of fasting) was specifically for the purification of the person that may be in sin or unclean. It is a day in which they were to afflict their souls (Lev 23:27, 32) by fasting (cf. Ezra 8:21) and repenting of one's sins (Ezek 18:30-31).

Richard Schwartz, Ph.D. points out "The laws of kashrut can lead to a reverence for life. Yet since the blood is the life of the body, Jews are forbidden to eat blood. 'For the life of the flesh is in the blood.' (Lev 17:11) By this verse alone some Jews may have been a vegetarian even during Passover. While most Jewish scholars assume that all Jews ate meat during the time that the Temple stood, it is significant that some (Tosafot, Yoma 3a, and Rabbeinu, Sukkah 42b) assert that even during the Temple period it was not an absolute requirement to eat meat."[233]

The prohibition against eating blood was extremely important and even foreigners were not exempt (Lev 12:10-12). There is always a tiny amount of blood even if the animals were drained of the blood. So the best way to stay pure and 'clean' was to avoid any animal meat that has blood in it, which basically means all land animal meats and meat products. The Torah Laws are to help us get back to a plant-based lifestyle that was found with Adam and Eve. The New Testament brings forth the new Adam and Eve, Jesus and his Blessed Mother Mary.

The teaching of the clean and the unclean was known in New Testament times as is indicated when Jesus used the parable of the dragnet to distinguish between the good fish and the bad fish as found in the Torah teaching on Kosher. "Once again, the kingdom of heaven is like a net that was let down into the lake and caught all kinds of fish. When it was full, the fishermen pulled it up on the shore. Then they sat down and collected the good fish in baskets, but threw the bad away." Mt 13:47, 48

Purification is a key biblical paradigm in both the Old and New Testament texts.
- Christianity began with the Aramaic phrase: "Purify thyself and believe the Good News." Mk 1:15
- "He has clean hands and a pure heart." Psalms 24:4
- "I have made my heart clean. I am pure." Prov 20:9
- "Blessed are the pure in heart," Matt 5:8

- "Purify your hearts."   James 4:8
- "Seeing ye have purified your souls." 1 Peter 1:22
- "thou will show thyself pure." 2 Samuel 22:27; Psalm 18;26
- "He shall purify himself." Num 19:12
- "many shall be purified and made white." Dan 12:10
- "Every word of God is pure." Prov. 30:5
- "Purifying himself." Acts 21:26;
- "Sanctified to the purifying of the flesh." Heb 9:13
- "Keep thyself pure ..." 1 Tim 5:22
- "Unto the pure all things are pure;" Titus 1:15
- "The wisdom that is from above is first pure." Ja 3:17

As the famous 5th century monk Dionysius the Areopagite says, "Purified souls, being raised up to the heights of contemplation, participate in the Divine, 'Thus do we learn that it is the Cause and Origin and Being and Life of all creation. (Gen 1) It is a Principle of Illumination to them that are being enlightened; a Principle of Perfection to them that are being perfected; a principle of Deity to them that are being deified; and of Simplicity to them that are being brought into simplicity.'[3]"[234]

D. A Toxicology Study on the Torah

A fascinating study by a researcher looking at Leviticus XI and Deuteronomy XIV, gives some scientific support for God's wisdom. "Much of the wisdom in the Divine Design for meats was confirmed by a 1953 study in which Dr. David Macht of Johns Hopkins University reported the toxic effects of animal flesh on a controlled growth culture."[235] "His results show that the lower the growth percentage of the culture, the more toxic the flesh.

---

[3] Illumination: as in Purgation, Illumination and Union. Perfection: technical usage as in 1 Cor. 2:6; Phil. 3:15. Deity: as St. Bernard bluntly says: "To experience this state is to be deified." Simplicity: soul turns from complex world to having one desire - for God, in a simple and unified state, Mat 6:22.

Note that the flesh of animals and fish given to us by God for food are all nontoxic, but all forbidden animals lie in the toxic range."[236]

"His results show that the lower the growth percentage of the culture, the more toxic the flesh. Note that the flesh of animals and fish given to us by God for food are all nontoxic, but all forbidden animals lie in the toxic range." Animals without percentage rankings in the chart were not studied, but are included here to provide a more comprehensive list of clean and unclean meats. "Don't get confused! Any number above 75 percent is nontoxic, or clean."[237]

Quadrupeds (Four Footed)
Clean (Cloven-hoofed and cud chewing) - calf (82%); deer (98%); goat (90%); ox (91%); sheep (94%).

Unclean - black bear (59%); camel (41%); cat (62%); guinea pig (46%); dog (62%); fox (58%); grizzly bear (55%); ground hog (53%); hamster (46%); horse (39%); opossum (53%); rabbit (49%); rat (55%); rhinoceros (60%); squirrel (43%); swine (54%).

Birds
Clean - goose (85%); chicken (83%); coot (88%); duck (98%); pigeon (93%); quail (89%); swan (87%); turkey (85%).
Unclean - bat; cormorant; crow (46%); eagle; falcon; hawk; heron; ibis; kite; nighthawk; osprey; ostrich; owl (62%); pelican; raven red-tail hawk (36%); sparrow hawk (63%); sea gull; stork, vulture.

Fish
Clean (with scales and fins) - black bass (80%); black drum (105%); bluefish (80%); carp (90%); channel bass (80%); chub (91%); cod (98%); croaker (90%); flounder (83%); flying fish (87%); goldfish (88%); haddock (80%); hake (98%); halibut (82%); herring (100%); kingfish (83%); mullet (87%); pike (98%); pompano (110%); porgy (80%); rainbow trout (81%); rock bass (100%); salmon (81%); smelt

(90%); sea bass (103%); shad (100%); Spanish mackerel (98%); spot (80%); sturgeon (87%); tuna (88%); white perch (81%); carolina whiting (84%); yellow perch 87%).

Unclean (without scales and fins) - catfish (48%); clams; crabs; eel (40%); lobster; octopus; oysters; porcupine fish (60%); puffer (51%); sand skate (59%); scallops; shark (62%); shrimp; squid; stingray (46%); toad fish (49%).

Basic science would indicate that animals who eat other animals would have a higher toxic percentage then animals who ate leaves and grass (which have chlorophyll a blood purifier). Animals store toxins and poisons in their fat cells and organs and the more animals, other animals eat, the higher the toxin rate in their cells. The Biblical Jews on the subject of kosher were in line with the modern biochemistry and toxicology!

In the Old Testament, the dietary principles of a pure diet (Kosher) are basically that they are allowed to eat the "clean" vegetarian animals (sheep, goat, ox, etc.) and not allowed to eat the 'unclean' meat eating animals (lions, bears, wolves, etc.) or the scavenger animals (pigs, wild boars, sharks, clams, shrimp, etc.). God was showing his people which meats were safe and which meats were unsafe, from the biblical teachings. The unclean are connected to sin and evil that can come upon the people as with Numbers 11. Another obvious text: "Do not make yourself detestable with all these crawling beasts; do not defile yourself with them, do not be defiled by them; 'For it is I, Yahweh, who am your God.' You have been sanctified and have become holy because I am holy; do not defile yourself with all these beasts that crawl on the ground." Lev 11:43, 44

E. Early Writers on the Essenes

Josephus and Philo were Jewish scholars and historians whose writings were around New Testament times.

A New Testament use of the Essenes is found as the Scribes, a religious party. "In Gospel material formulated relatively late, the scribes are independently named alongside the Pharisees (Mark 7:1, 5; Matt. 5:20; 12:38; 15:1; 23:2; Luke 5:21; 6:7; 11:53; 15:2; John 8:3) and are therefore reckoned as a group to be distinguished from the latter. On the other hand, there were occasionally "Scribes who belonged to the Pharisee party" (Mark 2:16; cf. John 3:1-12; 7:50-52; 19:39) and perhaps also scribes who were members of none of the great religious parties. In any case, the group designation 'scribes' strongly suggest the thought of the Essenes as the elite group in Judaism at that time, even after the destruction of the Temple. The oldest of our Gospels independently names, alongside the Pharisees, also the Herodians (Mark 3:6; 12:13; cf. 8:15; Matt. 22:16)."[238]

The name that Jesus was commonly known was "Jesus the Nazorean"[4] and also "Jesus the Nazarene"[5]. The term Nazarene describes a person who came from the town of Nazareth, which Jesus did.[6] The Nazarites were a branch of the Essenes and about 16 times Jesus is referred to as in this manner of a Nazarite or a Nazorean, directly relating him to the Essenes, put simply Jesus was an Essene.

The Nazoreans (Ac 24:5; cf. Ac 24:14, 28:22); the Sadducees (Ac 5:17), the Pharisees (Ac 15:5, 26:5) and the Essenes (Josephus: *The Life* 2 sec.10) are all characterized as 'Sects' of Judaism. The writers who mentioned the Essenes are: Philo, Pliny, Dio Chrysostom, Josephus, Hippolytus and Epiphanius. Josephus claims to have spent time with the

---

[4] (Mt 2:23; 26:71: Lk 18:37; Jn 18:5, 7; 19:19; Ac 2:22; 3:6; 4:10; 6:14; 22:8; 26:9; cf. 9:5)

[5] (Mk 1:24; 10:47; 14:67; 16:6; Lk 4:34; 24:19)

[6] (Mt 21:11; Jn 1:45-46; Ac 10:38; cf. Mk 1:9; Lk 4:16)

Essenes at age 16 (ca. 53-54 CE). Josephus writes about three "Jewish philosophical schools" in this period: the Sadducees, the Pharisee's and the Essenes.[239]

Josephus says of the Essenes, "they were stricter than all Jews in not undertaking work on the seventh day" and they held Moses in greatest reverence.[240] They were very interested in the study of the "holy books" and other ancient writings in order to "search out medicinal roots and the properties of stones" to heal diseases.[241] The Essenes held angels in importance and they also gave prophecy in the community. And the Essenes believed in bodily resurrection,[242] and in everlasting life,[243] and in Messianic Apocalypse.[244] Philo says they ate "bread and vegetables".

"The Hebrew word for 'meat' (basar) was explained by the Talmudists with the following acronym: bet: shame, sin: corruption, resh: worms. The more flesh, the more worms." [245] This school of thought in the biblical Jewish tradition connects meat directly with sin.

Kosher food was of great importance for the Essenes and most of the early sects of Judaism. It was so important that they would die for it. "Philo reports that Jewish women were offered 'swine's flesh' and tortured if they refused to eat it during anti-Jewish riots in Alexandria ca. 38 C.E."[246]

"According to Josephus, the Romans tortured the Essenes during the first Jewish revolt (66-74 C.E.) for refusing to renounce the dietary rules: 'They were racked and twisted, burnt and broken, and made to pass through every instrument of torture in order to induce them to blaspheme their lawgiver and to eat some forbidden thing. Yet, they refused to yield to either demand, nor even once did they cringe to their persecutors or shed a tear. Smiling in their agonies, mildly deriding their tormentors, they cheerfully resigned their souls, confident that they would receive them back again."[247]

Josephus refers to a certain company of Jewish priests who "being truly pious towards God supported themselves on figs and nuts," a reference to a vegetarian diet that was an Essene custom.[248]   Jesus was a Nazarite (from Joseph) and Mary was an Essene from her mother Joachim and Anne, (confirmed by mystic Anne Catherine Emmerick's visions in her books) they were part of the larger Essene community.

"Fasting was a regular Jewish custom, observed by the reforming sects also (cf. Mark 2:18). The duty of observing the 'day of fast' is mentioned in Qumran document CD 6:19, along with 'distinguishing between clean and unclean, making known between the holy and the profane, observing the Sabbath according to its interpretation and the feasts....'"[249]

The Qumran disciplines were an attempt at a radical transformation of the human condition to a healthier and holier state of life. Part of this effort to become "another man" (1 Sam 10:6) is the experience of ecstasy and other uplifted states of consciousness. Ecstatic behavior was often associated with prophecy. (1 Sam 10:5-13) Prophecy was part of the Essenes as noted by Josephus[250] and the Therapetae were noted by Philo for their strong ecstatic element. The prophets were credited with miracles and healing diseases (1 Kgs 17:10-24; 2 Kgs 4:8-37; Isa 38:1-8; Num 21:6-9). Jesus was also thought to be a prophet because of his healing miracles as in Mark 1:27; 6:2-4, 14-15, etc. The Essenes were also known for their healing arts.

Rabbi Gabriel Cousens, MD an expert on the Essenes notes that "According to Philo and other authors of that time the Essenes were vegetarians (also confirmed by modern historians such as Robert Eisenman, PhD) and took no drink other than rainwater or the juice of fruits. It is said that their diet was fruits, vegetables, nuts, seeds, and grains."[251]

F. Christianity a Continuation of the Essenes

One scholar of the Dead Sea Scrolls, Upton Ewing, in his book, *The Prophet of the Dead Sea Scrolls,* gives a rather convincing set of reasons on this topic. "Accordingly, so-called 'Palestinian Christianity' can be better understood historically as a continuation of, rather than an outgrowth of so-called 'Essenism.' The seven points which further illustrate this to be true are as set forth in the following premises:"[252]

(1) "That these devoutly religious people were the only ones in their part of the world whose common custom was evidenced by the wearing of a single white garment.

(2) That they were the only sect in their part of the world who practiced an economy whereby everything was held in common.

(3) That they were the only people in their part of the world whose religious leaders, or priesthood, practiced celibacy.

(4) That they were the only sect in their part of the world who opposed the custom of slavery.

(5) That they were the only religious sect, not alone in their own country but in the entire Roman world, who opposed the custom of animal sacrifice.

(6) That they were the only people in Palestine or of the greater Roman world who opposed the slaughter of animals for food.

(7) That they were the only people of Palestine and the outside Roman world whose way of life was opposed to war and the soldier' calling."[253]

All of these groups lived in the same general area of Galilee and the Dead Sea, in a way they were neighboring towns and villages. They were all orthodox Jews with basically the same Jewish beliefs and practices. As neighbors and friends they all interacted and may have even worked and worshiped together at times. There is no indication in the literature that these groups (Essenes, Nazarenes,

Therapeutae) had differences with one another but there is indication that these groups were at odds with the Pharisees and Sadducees in Jerusalem. These groups were really one large group of closely associated sects such that they were one sect, different branches on the same tree. And the trunk of that tree could be called the Essenes. This is the community that Jesus and Mary grew up in.

Rabbi Gabriel Cousens, MD a modern day Jewish Essene, gives some good insight.[254] ; "The Essene Archetype is a very intriguing, inspiring ideal. The ancient Essenes were historically recognized as the mystical Jewish prophets of the desert. They considered themselves, in their terms, 'the holy ones of God'. It is no accident that the term *Essene* comes from the Northern Aramaic word *chasya*, which means *saint* in Greek, which was the way they were perceived by the general population. From the time of Hannokh they were also known as *B'nei Aliyah*, the children of ascension. Many of the early Jewish followers of Jesus were also Essene; it is also strongly suggested historically that Mary's parents (Joachim and Anna), Jesus' parents (Mary and Joseph), his brother James, and John the Baptist were also Essene. In 2007, at an Easter talk,[255] Pope Benedict XVI acknowledged that the home where Jesus had his last meal was an Essene home, and his second volume of *Jesus of Nazareth* (2011) mentions the Essenes in general and in specific in the context of Jesus' 'Last Supper.'[256] This suggests that Jesus was clearly associated with the Essenes. If he was not formally trained as an Essene as some historians suggest, he was at least close to them in some spiritual and lifestyle alignment. The Essene existence is first mentioned about 500 B.C., after the fall of the First Temple in 586 B.C., in Pythagora's biography, where he studied with them on Mt. Carmel and came down enlightened and as a teacher of live foods [raw vegans]. These were called the Galilean Essenes of the north, where Jesus came from. The Galilean Essenes were also given the name Nazarenes, as was Jesus."[257]

Rabbi Cousens, "The Essenes lived in various communities all over the Middle East. They totaled in number between 4,000 to 10,000 people. This included the Qumran Essene community, which began in 186 B.C. near the Dead Sea. There were also Essenes at the Sea of Galilee, Mt. Carmel, in Egypt at Lake Mareotis, as well as in the areas that are now known as Lebanon and Damascus. These Essene groups, which resided all over the region, had slightly different styles according to the local culture, but shared the basics of Essene life and spirituality. They believed in creating a lifestyle that would support the human transformation into a whole and healthy life. They were noted by the historian Philo, for their focus on living ecstatically. They lived strictly and honorably by these ethics. Historical evidence indicates that the vast majority of the Essenes adhered to a plant-source-only and/ or live-foods diet."[258]

F. James the Second Pope was Vegetarian

James, a servant of God and of the Lord Jesus Christ (1.1), as the author of the *Epistle of James*, is not one of the twelve but the cousin of Jesus (Gal 1:19), and the administrator of the Jerusalem community (Ac 12:17). He played a leading role in the apostolic Council (Acts 15:13-21) forming the early Christian community. After Paul's third missionary journey they spoke in Jerusalem before Paul's arrest (Ac 21:17-25).

Peter was the first Bishop of the Church for a short time. After being rescued by the angel he had to flee the city. Then James took over as the head of the Jerusalem Church and of all that was first Christians. James, for two to three decades was the head of the early Church and in some ways the Bishop to both Peter and Paul. As the leader, James was clearly the undisputed successor to Jesus and certainly was 'the Bishop of Bishops' or 'Archbishop'. James is mentioned not only in the Gospels but also named or implied in other early writings from the Church Fathers, notably Origen, Eusebius, Epiphanisus, Hegesippus and Jerome.

Also in some texts that are not accepted as part of the canon of Catholic Church books but historically they still have importance include: the *Gospel of Hebrews*, the *Gospel of Nazoraeans*, and the *Gospel of the Ebionites, Gnostic Gospel of Thomas*, the Pseudoclementine writings and the Apocryphal Gospel the *Protevangelium of James*. All this is important and James was an important figure in the very beginning of the Christian Church.

"According to the early Christian historian Hegesippus (2nd cent.), who is excerpted in Eusebius' *Ecclesiastical History*, 'James, the brother of the Lord, succeeded to the government of the Church in conjunction with the apostles. He has been called the Just by all from the time of our Savior to the present day for there were many called James. He was holy from his mother's womb and he drank no wine nor strong drink, nor did he eat flesh. No razor came upon his head; he did not anoint himself with oil, and he did not use the bath. He alone was permitted to enter into the holy place for he wore not woolen but linen garments...'"[259]

Yes, James the second Pope, "drank no wine nor strong drink, nor did he eat flesh" he was a vegetarian. He followed the kosher laws and Torah laws exactly which leads a person to be a vegetarian. He also knew Jesus and Mary and probably followed their example since they were model vegetarians.

H. Essene Community of the New Covenant

Joseph Cardinal Ratzinger (who became Pope Benedict XVI) was the Prefect of the Congregation for the Doctrine of the Faith and he along with the Pontifical Biblical Commission (2001) released a document: *The Jewish People and Their Sacred Scriptures in the Christian Bible*, it speaks several times of the Essenes. They connect the Essene community with the new covenant school of thought: "the Qumran group formed the community of the new covenant."[260]

The Commission makes the connection between the Essenes and the Christian message; and point out that the theology of Jesus is closer to the Essenes. "His belief in angels and the resurrection of the body, as well as the eschatological expectation attributed to him in the Gospels, is much closer to the theology of the Essenes and the Pharisees."[261] Whereas Cardinal Joseph Ratzinger stopped short of stating that Jesus was an Essene, he did state later as Pope Benedict in his book, *Jesus of Nazareth*,[262] "The earnest religiosity of the Qumran writings is moving; it appears that not only John the Baptist, but possibly Jesus and his family as well, were close to the Qumran community. At any rate, there are numerous points of contact with the Christian message in the Qumran writings. It is a reasonable hypothesis that John the Baptist lived for some time in this community and received part of his religious formation from it."[263] The weight of the evidence is that Jesus was an Essene and they were a kosher or kosher vegetarian Jewish community, the forerunner of Christian communities.

There is only one mention of the Virgin Mary in the Acts of the Apostles, after the ascension they returned to Jerusalem. "Together they devoted themselves to constant prayer. There were some women in their company, and Mary the mother of Jesus, and his brethren." Acts 1:14 Then at Pentecost it is written, "All were filled with the Holy Spirit" and "They devoted themselves to the apostle's instruction and the communal life, to the breaking of bread and the prayers. A reverent fear overtook them all, for many wonders and signs were performed by the Apostles." Ac 2:4, 42, 43.

Mary the mother of Jesus was involved in the beginning of the Jerusalem Community. This community was centered in Jerusalem but was scattered in towns and villages around Jerusalem and throughout Galilee; whether she lived in Jerusalem or more likely in one of the neighboring towns or back in her home town of Nazareth, she would have been part of the Jerusalem community, their beliefs and practices. The Kosher orientation of the Jerusalem community was one of their main Jewish practices. Mary the Mother of Jesus would have been kosher all this time. Some mystics (i.e. either Blessed Anne Catherine Emmerick, Venerable Mary of Agreda; St. Bridget of Sweden; or St. Elizabeth of Schoenau.[264] on the following quote) describe the Virgin Mary as a vegetarian. "She ate very sparingly and took no meat, though she prepared it for Joseph. She usually ate cooked vegetables and bread, fruit and fish."[265]

Joseph Cardinal Ratzinger became Pope in 2005. In Pope Benedict XVI book *Jesus of Nazareth*,[266] he writes on the possible community connections of the family of Jesus: "An accidental discovery after the Second World War led to excavation at Qumran, which brought to light texts that some scholars have associated with yet another movement known until then only from literary references: the so-called Essenes. This group had turned its back on the Herodian temple and its worship to withdraw to the Judean desert. There it created monastic-style communities, but also a religiously motivated common life for families. It also established a productive literary center and instituted distinctive rituals, which included liturgical ablutions and common prayers. The earnest religiosity of the Qumran writings is moving. It appears that not only John the Baptist, but possibly Jesus and his family as well, were close to the Qumran community. At any rate, there are numerous points of contact with the Christian message in the Qumran writings. It is a reasonable hypothesis that John the Baptist lived for some time in this community and received part of his religious formation from it."[267]

In Acts 6:7 we read: "The word of God continued to spread, while the same time the number of the disciples in Jerusalem enormously increased. There were many priests among those who embraced the faith." Who were these many priests who embraced the faith? Surely they were not the Pharisees and Sadducees! This means that these priests

who embraced the faith were from the Essene community:
the Essenes, the Therapeutae and the Nazarites and others all
under the umbrella of the Essenes.

The Essenes seemed to have disappeared a century or
so after Jesus death and at the same time the followers of 'the
Way' Christianity grew enormously during this same time
period. Jesus spent only a week or two in Jerusalem and
nearly all of his time in the greater Galilee area where the
Essenes were located, around 4,000 of them, yet another
estimate has been around 10,000, it depends on how much
the sects are included in the count. Perhaps many of these
converts to Christianity came from the Essenes, Therapeutae
and the Nazarenes, who were all looking for the coming of
the Messiah. Perhaps this is why the Essenes disappeared a
century after Jesus death because most if not all of them
became the first Christians!

I. The First Jewish-Christian Communities
Considered Jesus a Vegetarian

Professor Kalechofsky, PhD writes: "With the fall of
Jerusalem in 70 C.E. came the destruction of the Temple and
the disappearance of priestly slaughterers. "Above all, an
enormous sense of mourning must have hung over the
surviving remnant. A mourner loses his appetite and his
interest in the joys of living. For the expression of these
feelings, a number of mourners must have been attracted to
the ascetic cults of ancient Israel, which had already existed
for quite some time before the destruction. The Qumran
group associated with the Dead Sea Scrolls appears to have
already disappeared, but there were others - Nazirites,
Rechabites, Essenes, Therapeutae, and Zakokites. With the
destruction of the Temple, the ascetic cults must have
expressed as never before a predominant mood of the people.
A central feature of some of these ascetic groups was
abstinence from the eating of meat. Celibacy, fasting, and
other forms of privation also marked the ascetic regimen, but

vegetarianism was a prominent symbol of the ascetic life, and was now fittingly associated with mourning for the destruction of the Temple."[268] "Following the destruction of the Temple, the number of recluses who would not eat meat or drink wine increased in Israel."[269]

Some orthodox Jewish writers recognize that in order to fulfill the laws of the Torah the vegetarian lifestyle was the ideal.[270] All of these groups lived in the same general area of Galilee, Nazareth, and the Dead Sea. They all had similar beliefs and practices, they were neighbors and friends. Jesus lived with, ate with, preached too and taught many of these early communities.

These early Jewish communities sought out a life of purification and healing through fasting, a plant-based kosher diet, and a pure lifestyle. For the early Jewish communities the Essenes, Nazirites, Rechabites, Essenes, Therapeutae, and Zakokites, a Kosher lifestyle and for some kosher vegetarianism and fasting were a way of life. (Nazirites cited in Ac 24:5, 14; 28:22)

Therefore we see that certain early Christian communities the Encratites, Ebionites, Marcionites, Manichaeans, Priscillianists, also emphasized the importance of purification, a kosher diet and also vegetarianism and fasting which was part of their lifestyle. Some of them taught that Jesus was a vegetarian and that Jesus was a man of self-control and temperance. Love, Joy, Peace, Self-Control, Temperance (Gal 5:23; 1 Cor 7:9, 9:25); These are fruits of the Spirit, Alleluia! (Ti 1:8; 2 Pt 1:6) People today need to be "given instruction in the Way of the Lord." (Acts 18:25)

In the *Encyclopedia of the Early Church*, the Church Fathers[271] wrote that certain groups abstained from particular foods including: the Encratites, Ebionites, Marcionites, Manichaeans, and Priscillianists, who seem to have considered Jesus a vegetarian.[272] This is very significant to have early Christian communities believing this.

"Origen says that these Jews who have received Jesus Christ were all called by the name 'Ebionites'"[273] And St. Epipanius (ca. 350) writes that "the Ebionite Sect was in existence (35 CE)."[274] Bishop Epiphanius (A.D. 315-403) of Constantia in Cyprus, in his book *Panarion*[275] states, 'Whenever you speak to them (Ebionites) concerning flesh food, the Ebionites reply they were vegetarian because "Christ revealed it to me.'[276] This is another reference connecting the Ebionites to the early Christians.

According to the *Encyclopedia of the Dead Sea Scrolls* it writes: "In the second and third centuries, the Church Fathers Irenaeus (c. 130-200 CE), Clement of Alexandria (c. 150-215 CE) and Hippolytus (c. 170-236 CE) applied that name Encratites to a diverse array of early Christian groups adopting ascetic practices such as celibacy, abstinence from wine, and vegetarianism. Particularly important is an organized Jewish-Christian community that, according to Irenaeus,[277] was founded in the latter part of the second century in Mesopotamia by Tatian.

Tatian was a pupil of Justin Martyr (c. 100-165 CE) and author of the Diatessaron (a famous harmony of the four canonical Gospels). Justin Martyr was involved in Christianity during the beginning of the early Church and surely would have known the Apostle John. The Encratite community that Tatian founded was vegetarian which means that Justin was probably a vegetarian himself or at least approved of it.

This is significant to have this witness on vegetarianism so close to the original Christian community in Jerusalem. The connection here is important. Tatian was a disciple of Justin Martyr. Justin was probably a disciple of the Apostle John or of one of his disciples, and John took care of Mary, which implies that perhaps Justin, John and Mary were vegetarian or at least approved of it!

The Virgin Mary and Jesus lived among these people for probably 25 years, assuming they were in Egypt for only five years, where they probably would have been associated with the Jewish Essene community called the Therapeutae in Egypt, who were versed in the healing arts. Then when Jesus started his ministry, the majority of the time he spent in this greater area of Galilee, except for the short times he spent preaching in Jerusalem. Thus Jesus was preaching to and eating with many of the people in these Jewish sects: the Nazarene's, the Essenes, the Ebionites, the Therapeutae's and others who were strict kosher and even vegetarian. In addition, almost all of his disciples and followers came from these groups, which were mostly or totally vegetarian. And those after Jesus time, continued with the vegetarian tradition, such as the Titan community mentioned above.

In the *Encyclopedia of the Early Church*, (1992) it mentions that the Church Fathers[278] had some good insights into fasting. The Christian fasts spiritually by abstaining from evil,[279] observing the commandments, confiding in God and serving him with a pure heart; fasting from food will help the poor: 'on the day of the fast, eat only bread and water and, working out the cost of the food you would have consumed, give a corresponding sum to a widow, an orphan, a needy person'.[280] The whole family will take part with joy: 'Observe these things with your children and all your household: thus you will be happy".[281]

Abstinence is a partial fast, esp. from meat and wine, which allows us to survive and hence to fast again.[282] It is ascesis, not aversion to diabolical foods.[283] Certain groups abstained from particular foods: Encratites, Ebionites, Marcionites, Manichaeans, Priscillianists, who seem to have considered Jesus a vegetarian.[284] Some claimed that St Peter "ate only bread, olives and herbs"[285].

155

One of the primary reasons that these Jewish people in community became vegetarian and upheld it was to fulfill the teachings of the Torah, God's Word. In Mosaic Law, blood must be strictly separated from food. (Lev 3:17; 7:26-27; 17:3-7; 10B14; 19:26; Deut 12:15-16, 20-28; 15:19-23; 1 Sam 14:32-35; Ex 33:25) The prohibition against eating blood was extremely important and even foreigners were not exempt (Lev 12:10-12). The easy way, in fact the only way to truly fulfill this requirement was to be vegetarian and not eat any meat that has blood in it.

J. The Divine Life is the Culture of Life

There is a Divine Life that we are called to which requires purification and gives a richness of life. The word "eternal" is only found two or three times in the Old Testament but is found about 45 times in the new. John uses this word more than any other (the Synoptic, in Paul, and in the letters). The common translation from the Greek is 'eternal' yet another translation is 'divine' most of the time the translation is talking about the here and now, not the future after we die. Divine is actually a better translation in many ways then eternal because divine indicates a present action, place or thing, 'in the now'. Jesus talked about the kingdom of God as present among us, now!

'Eternal life' or 'Divine life' is found throughout the New Testament; Mt 19.16, 25.46; Mk 10.17, 10.30; Lk 10.25,18.18; Jn 3.15, 4.36, 5.39, 6.54, 6.68, 10.28, 12.25, 17.2, 17.3; Acts 13.48; Rom 2.7, 5.21, 6.23; 2 Cor (4.17), 4.18; 1 Ti 6.12, 6.19; (2 Ti 2.10); Titus 1.2, 3.7; (Heb 5.9, 6.2, 9.12, 9.14, 9.15); 1 Pet 5.10); 1 Jn 1.2, 2.25, 3.15, 5.11, 5.13, 5.20; Jude (1.7, 1.21). The verses in parentheses have a different emphasis or word, than life.

The key verse here is 2 Peter 1.3, 4: "That divine power of his has freely bestowed on us everything necessary for a life of genuine piety, through knowledge of him who called us by his own glory and power. By virtue of them he has bestowed on us the great and precious things he promised, so that through these you who have fled a world corrupted by lust might become sharers of the divine nature." This Divine Life is part of the Culture of Life that brings purification and also richness into our lives through the things that we do, eating is one of them.

The Christian is striving to move away from the world, the flesh and the devil; and towards the Kingdom of Heaven, which is among us as Divine Life. We are involved in a choice; the Culture of Life vs. the culture of death. Pope John Paul II brought this terminology to the forefront, especially in his encyclical: *Gospel of Life*.

> "For us too, Moses' invitation rings out loud and clear: 'See, I have set before you this day life and prosperity, death and disaster' (Deut 30:15 JB) . . . 'This invitation is very appropriate for us who are called day by day to the "daily duty" of choosing between the "culture of life" and the "culture of death".'" "The Gospel of Life is at the heart of Jesus' message." "Jesus says: 'I came that they may have life, and have it abundantly' (Jn 10:10)."
> Blessed Pope John Paul II - March 25, 1995,
> The Encyclical: *Gospel of Life*, versus 28, 1.

The pilgrimage in the Culture of Life needs to recognize the importance of the penitential diet and fasting, which have been around for over 3,700 years in biblical times to the present; they are both purification methods. In the Bible the penitential diet is basically the kosher diet, it is considered a pure diet.

Rabbi Jesus in the New Testament never rejected the purification of the body and soul but in fact encouraged it, such as with his 40 day fast. Fasting and the kosher diet or a penitential diet was the number one method of purification of the body in the Bible, and also in the Christian hermits, monks and penitents throughout the centuries. A penitential diet takes out certain foods that are not considered healthy.

In the Old Testament the Jewish people lived a simple lifestyle and they had three main altars that bring life, that were sacred to them.

- The first is the sacred altar of sacrifice; this was the forerunner of the Eucharistic table.
- The second the sacred altar was the altar of the marriage bed which brings forth new life in children.
- The third sacred altar was the kitchen table, since it brings forth life through health and avoiding sickness. At the kitchen table they only served kosher foods, kosher means 'pure' and pure foods imply that it is life-giving. All Jews at that time were kosher; it was part of who they were.[286]

The first Christian community in Jerusalem was the new Eden building upon the first Eden. The practical concrete biblical emphasis of these early Christian-Jews lifestyle was meant to be a life of purification to grow in holiness and purity of heart. The early Church and even today in Christian Churches the emphasis on community was central. The Culture of Life implies a culture, and to live and thrive in that culture implies some type of community. The dietary emphasis in this book works best in a community setting for the support and sharing of the lifestyle.

Spiritual Nutrition involves the physiological, the biochemical, the psychological and the spiritual, which are intimately intertwined; they grow unto perfection and holiness as one being. We are called to be, Healthy, Happy, and Holy unto God: in our body, soul and spirit. This means being rich in Sacred Sensuousness, the delight in the senses, including the sense of smell and taste and touch, in sensual enjoyment, in sensuousness as a proper religious attitude and a spiritual experience of the Good News; which comes to us first through our holy senses. "Our message concerns that which was from the beginning. We have heard it; we have seen it with our own eyes; we have looked at it and our hands have touched it: the life-giving Word ... so that your joy may be complete." 1 Jn 1:1-4. A life rooted in sensuousness thrives whereas a life entangled in sensuality gets wrapped up in sensual pleasure, it never finds full joy and it chokes and withers.

Sacred Sensuousness is "walking in the light" (1 Jn 1:7) of the enjoyment of our senses. This is bringing us closer to a personal transformation to Jesus Christ sensuousness, to His enjoyment of His Father's earthly creation, and to the present day cultures activities of kosher foods, vegetarian foods, raw foods, live foods, feasting, fasting, festivals, dancing, music and other Ways of Beauty! St. Irenaeus an early Church Father stated; "The glory of God is the human being fully alive."

Jesus and Mary were both fully human. God shares his Divine nature (2 Pet 1:4) with us, His fellow heirs. (Rom 8:16-17). The purpose of purification of the body, soul and spirit is as Jesus stated; "That they may have life, life in abundance." Jn 10:10

"My dear friend, I hope you are in good health and may you thrive in all other ways as you do in the spirit." 3 John 2

K. Purification and Consecration

The early Christians had commitments, covenants and consecrations; they were a communal body a community of one mind and heart (Acts 1) bound together to purify themselves and their relationships. There are many types of consecrations by various authors. One of the most famous is St. Luis De Montfort who wrote about a 33 day consecration to Jesus Christ through Mary which is composed of various prayers, devotions and meditations.

Joaquin Alonso in his book, *Fatima Message and Consecration* (1984), writes about personal consecration (for one person or a few people) and social consecration (parish, diocese, communities or a nation) and also Sacramental Consecration: "At this point a distinction arises which I deem pertinent. There is a Sacramental Consecration, and there are others which we could call Devotional Consecrations, if we give to this word devotion all its force."[287]

Fr. Alonso continues, "Our reflection would remain incomplete without a clear reference to the Church, the People of the New Alliance. It is in the light of the Covenant, actually, that consecration can be fully understood. It is then that God consecrates his People and that they give themselves to the Lord: 'If you hold fast to my covenant . . . you shall be my very own, a consecrated nation' – Yahweh proclaims to the Hebrews at the time of sealing with them, through the mediation of Moses, the Covenant at Sinai (Ex 19.5-6). And Christ Jesus, in immolating himself as a victim in the sacrifice of the New Covenant, addressing his Father in the Cenacle before his disciples, declares these words which were cited by John Paul II in the Act of Consecration at Fatima: 'And for their sake I consecrate myself so that they too may be consecrated in truth.' (Jn 17, 19). The phrase used by Jesus can also be translated in this manner: 'For their sake I sanctify myself so that they too may be sanctified.'"[288]

The eminent French theologian Fr. Rene Laurentin gives a clear, factual and systematic outline of the events for the consecrations of Fatima in his book: *The Meaning of Consecration Today, a Marian Model for a Secularized Age* (1992). "The essence of the Christian life is to be found in consecration. God himself saw to this in order to effect the divinization of man. This is the reason why St. Paul called Christians 'the saints'. Incorporated in the body of Christ, which is the Church, Christians are necessarily consecrated to God; therefore, they are sanctified by God. In the New Covenant, Christians actually realize and embody the precept that was merely enunciated in the Old Testament: 'You shall be holy; for I the Lord your God am holy' (Lev 19:2; also 20:26). The saying of Jesus in the Gospel according to Matthew confirms this: "You therefore must be perfect as your heavenly Father is perfect" (Mt 5:48)."[289]

"Paul actually defined his own mission as an apostle as involving the finality of consecration men to God; this was for the sake of their divinization, for the Good News of the Gospels was announced in order to transform their lives in God. Paul wrote that he was "a minister of Christ Jesus to the Gentiles in the priestly service of the Gospel of God, so that the offering of the Gentiles may be acceptable, sanctified by the Holy Spirit" (Rom 15:16). Paul himself was the minister of this consecration, but each Christian thus consecrated had to offer his own life in a sacrifice of praise (cf. Rom 12:1; Phil 2:17, 4:18; Heb 13:15; 1 Pet 2:5)."[290]

The word "sacrifice" (*sacri-ficium*) means, etymologically, to make or render something sacred, that is, to "consecrate". "St. Augustine easily perceived the identity between "consecration", gift, and sacrifice: 'Man himself *consecrated* to the name of God and given over to God, is a sacrifice in the sense that he dies to the world in order to live for God. Sacrifice is the movement of man into God, the consummation of man in God; it involves a consecration of all the moments of one's life. As the Apostle Paul understood so well, it means offering up one's body "as a living sacrifice, holy and acceptable to God' (Rom 12:1; cf. Phil 2:17; Rom 1:9).'"[291]

To give an example of a national consecration by the Bishops of the world let us look at Fr. Rene Laurentin who writes that: "The most substantial segment of the whole consecration movement is the one in which some of the popes have controlled the universal Church, namely, the movement arising out of the revelation of Fatima. Our Lady asked, there, for the consecration of Russian by the pope. Lucia indicated that this request was first enunciated on July 13, 1917; she did not formally and explicitly bring it out until 1929, however. Eight Popes did different forms of consecrations and Pope John Paul II did one with all the bishops of the world in 1982 and 1984. Within one year after the 1984 consecrations a whole series of events took place. Just one year after the Consecration, in March of 1985, the President of the Soviet Union, Chernenko, died. Mikhail Gorbachev was made President. Gorbachev instituted *glasnost* and *perestroika* (freedom of the press and freedom of religion), which would lead to the downfall of Communism."[292] It was the events in the 1980's leading to the downfall of Communism in the early 1990's of which Pope John Paul II was definitely a part of the process. (See the authors' writings for a more detailed review of this.)

"Is it a surprise that *Jane's Defense Weekly*, quoted above, said that a nuclear war would probably have taken place in 1985? Or that Sister Lucia, who knew nothing of that report, said in the October 1993 interview: 'There would have been a nuclear war in 1985.'"[293] Sister Lucia was the visionary of Fatima that requested the consecration to Russia. This international consecration by the Pope probably saved the world from nuclear war in 1985, which shows the power of consecration on an international level. Think of what it can do on a personal level with your body!

Our personal pilgrimage in life involves seven dimensions that we exist in as we go up the mountain of the Lord. Our personal purification starts with our Body, Soul and Spirit. Next the dimension of purification expands to our family and social relationships. Along with these other dimensions our purification deepens with Nature (the Living Planet) and with the Saints (Communion of Saints of which Jesus and Mary are part of).

The seven dimensions of purification that a person matures into spiritually are thus summarized:

The seven-fold Purification Dimensions include:
1. Purification of the Body
    Mt 16:24; Lk 9:23; 1 Cor 9:27; 2 Cor 7:1; 3 John 2
2. Purification of the Soul
    Rom 12:2; Heb 4:12; Lk 1:46
3. Purification of the Spirit
    Matthew 5:3-10
4. Purification of Family Relationships
    Matthew 5:17-48
5. Purification of Social Relationships
    Matthew 6:1-7:12
6. Purification of the Relationship with
       the Living Planet
    Deut 20.19-20; Ps 24:1; Ps 145:9
7. Purification of the Relationship with
       the Communion of Saints
    Heb 11:10; 12:1;13:14; 2 Cor 3:18; Eph 4:1-6

Jesus, Mary and Joseph are part of this communion of Saints. There are over 10,000 canonized saints in the Catholic Church, and millions of saints in heaven that have not been named. All of these Saints had their own penitential life or life of purification. All of these Saints involved purification on all these levels, some focused on certain levels of purification more than others. The goal of all this purification is of course holiness. "Let us wash off all that can soil either body or spirit, to reach perfection of holiness in the fear of God." 2 Cor 7:1

Back to this book on Smoothies and Greens a 33 day consecration for purification would be helpful. Commit 33 days to making smoothies and drinking greens (orange and other colors too). Thus make a consecration of thirty three days to purify these seven dimensions in your life of; Living Green with Smoothies and Chlorophyll Rich Foods. This will be a life-changing experience. "Do not conform yourselves to this age but be transformed by the renewal of your mind, so that you may judge what is God's will, what is good, pleasing and perfect." Rom 12:2

See the author (Jim Tibbetts) book on a thirty-three day consecration for the purpose of purification. It uses this book as a basis for this 33-day consecration.

"May the God of peace make you perfect and holy; and may you all be kept safe and blameless, spirit, soul and body, for the coming of our Lord Jesus Christ. 1 Thess 5:23

X. Resources

A. Raw Vegan Uncook books

There are many good raw food books on the market here are a few of them. It is best to buy several different authors to see their take on raw foods, basically they are very similar because it is all primarily raw foods although some do a little heating or cooking in the 80/20 raw food line. Buy at least four or five raw Uncook books!

Eating without Heating
  Sergei and Valya Boutenko
Green for Life
  Victoria Boutenko
Raw Family Publishing
www.rawfamily.com
	Rainbow Green Live-Food
	Cuisine; Conscious Eating
	Gabriel Cousens, MD
	Patagonia, Arizona
	www.raw-food.com
	www.treeoflife.nu

Recipes for Life *The Hallelujah Diet* Rhonda Malkamus Hallelujah Acres Pub. www.hacres	*The Raw Food Revolution* *Diet*, Cherie Soria Brenda Davis, RD Vesanto Melina, MS, RD www.bookpubco.com

Angel Foods
Cherie Soria
Living Light International
www.Rawfoodchef.com
	Back to the House of Health
	  Shelley Redford Young
	  Robert Young, PhD
	www.thephmiracle.us

Health Cuisine Anna Maria Clement www.healthfulcommunications.com (Hippocrates Inst., Florida)	*Rawsome!* Brigitte Mars www.brigittemars.com
Live in Magic Aimee & Denny Perrin York, Maine www.aimeeslivinmagic.com	*Hooked on Raw* www.rawfoodinfo.com by Rhio Beso Entertainment New York, N.Y. 10013

Living Green with Juices and Smoothies Anne Marie & Jim Tibbetts www.jimtibbetts.com	*Vital Creations* Chad Sarno www.rawchef.org
Living on Live Food Alissa Cohen Kittery, Maine 03904 www.AlissaCohen.com	*Thank God for Raw* Julie Wandling Healthy4 Him Pub. www.hacres.com
The Raw Gourmet Nomi Shannon Alive Books	*LifeFood Recipe Book* Annie & David Jubb Jubbs Longevity, Inc. www.lifefood.com
Raw Charlie Trotter and Roxanne Klein www.tenspeed.com	*Raw the Uncook Book* Juliano www.juliano.com
Living Cuisine and, *The Balanced Plate* Renee Loux Underkoffler www.reneeloux.com	*The Raw Truth, the art of preparing Living Foods* Jeremy A. Safron www.tenspeed.com
The Raw Truth, the art of loving foods Jeremy A. Safron and Renee Underkoffler www.lovingfoods.com	*Elaine's Pure Joy Kitchen* *Raw, Living, Organic, Vegan* Elaine Love www.Purejoylivingfoods.com
Dr. J.G. Schnitzer *Schnitzer-Intensive Nutrition* *& Schnitzer-Normal Nutrition* Schnitzer Publishers, D-7742 St. Georgen Black Forest W. Germany www.doc-schnitzer.com	*Warming Up to Living Food Smoothies* Book Publishing Company *Smoothies and other scrumptious delights* Elyssa Markowitz Alive Books www.alive.com
I Am Grateful Recipes & Lifestyles *Café Gratitude* Terces Engelhart & Richard Slayen San Francisco, CA.	*Raw Food Made Easy* Jennifer Cornbleet www.healthy-eating.com Book Publishing Company

Eating in the Raw *The Raw 50* - latest book Carol Alt Clarkson Potter Publishers www.clarksonpotter.com	*Raw in Ten Minutes* Bryan Au www.rawinten.com
Dining in the Raw Rita Romano Kensington Publishing Co. www.kensingtonbooks.com	*The Gourmet Uncook Book* Elizabeth Baker ProMotion Publishing 800-231-1776
The Raw Food Primer Suzanne Alex Ferrara Council Oak Books	*Vibrant Living* James Levin, MD GLO, Inc. www.GLOinc.com
Vice Cream, over 70 sinfully *delicious dairy-free delights* Jeff Rogers Celestial Arts www.tenspeed.com	*Raw Foods for Busy People* Jordan Maerin rawfoodsforbusypeople.com
Dr. Norman Walker *Diet and Salad* Norwalk Press 107 N. Cortez - Suite 200 Prescott, Arizona 86301	*The Uncook Book* *The Gourmet Uncook Book* Elizabeth Baker ProMotion Publishing San Diego, CA 92122
Everday Wholesome *Eating...Raw* Kim Wilsom www.hacres.com	How We All Went Raw Charles, Coralanne & George Nungesser www.hacres.com
Everyday Raw *Raw Food Real World* Matthew Kenney www.gibbs_smith.com	*The 80/10/10 Diet* Douglas Graham Food n' Sport Press
Sunfood Cuisine Frederic Patenaude www.rawfood.com	*Uncooking with Jameth* *and Kim* Jameth & Kim Sheridan Healthforce Publishing www.healthforce.net

These books on the raw food lifestyle are recommended for those moving into the raw and living foods movement. There are other books on raw and living foods out in the market place but they have not been reviewed yet so are not included in this list. Some that have been reviewed have not been included mostly because they emphasize too much cooking. Buy at least four or five of these books. It is best to have a small library to work with in dealing with nutrition and the living foods lifestyle. Alleluia!

Green Powders

Most of the places that make Protein Powders also have Green powders but here is a list of a few, there are many. Most major health food stores have a selection of different green powders.

Green Powders	
Barley Max Hallelujah Acres www.hacres.com	**Perfect Food** Garden of Life www.gardenoflife.com
Wheat Grass Powder, **Green Superfood** Amazing Grass www.amazinggrass.com	**Kyo Green** Wakunaga of America www.kyo-green.com www.kyolic.com
MacroGreens Macro Life Naturals www.macrogreens.com	**Chlorella** Jarrow Formulas www.jarrow.com
Green Magma Green Foods, Dr. Hagiwara www.greenfoods.com	**DocBroc's Power Plants** Dr. Robert Young www.phmiracleliving.com
Vitamineral Green Jameth Sheridan, ND www.healthforce.com	**Green Vibrance** Vibrant Health www.vibranthealth.us

Plant-based Protein Powders

The following are different plant-based protein powders from different companies in 2009-2011. I (Jim) have tried each one of these over the last few years, some I prefer more than others and some have better high quality protein combinations, but they are all good.

As a rule: **Avoid all Whey protein powders these are milk based.** There are a lot of milk and some animal based protein powders that should be avoided. Eat only non-animal, vegan, plant-based protein powders.

This section is a listing of different plant-based protein powders that are available. You can look them up and compare them and decide which is best for you. It is sometimes hard to find what you want in a health food store but online they are all available and the web address is given for each.

What is recommended by this author is to always use two different protein powders from two different companies. Different protein powders have different combinations of amino acids. Even though any one protein powder is adequate, two different protein powders from two different companies is an insurance that you will be getting all the amino acids needed in their right combination. The reason for using two different companies is because different companies process protein powder differently. Is one way better than the other, probably yes, but we don't know that, comparative analysis research on this question is yet to be done.

Various Types Vegan Protein Powders

Mixed Vegan Protein Powders	
Garden of Life **Raw Protein** Ingredients Raw Organic Sprout Blend: brown rice, amaranth, quinoa, millet, buckwheat, garbanzo bean, kidney bean, lentil, flax seed, adzuki bean, sunflower seed, pumpkin seed, chia seed, sesame seed. Serving size 22 g. 1 level scoop Protein 18 g 35% Garden of Life 5500 Village Blvd. West Palm Beach, FL 33407 www.gardenoflife.com	**Vegan Complete Whole Food** **Health Optimizer** **Natural flavor, berry flavor** The Thrive Diet, Brendan Brazier triathlete is the formulator of Vega products. www.brendanbrazier.com Ingredients Organic Hemp protein, organic yellow pea protein, organic brown rice protein, whole flax seed, natural vanilla flavor, xanthan gum, stevia leaf. (measure from maca root) Serving size 61 g. (2 scoops) Protein 28 g 52% Sequel Naturals, Ltd. Vancouver, BC V3C 6G5 866-839-8863

Vibrant Health
Pure Green Protein
Mixed berry
Ingredients
Yellow pea protein, alfalfa
protein, rice protein, spirulina
powder
Serving size   29.79 g. (1
        scoops, or 1 ounce)
Protein   20 g
Formulated and distributed by:
Vibrant Health
Canaan, CT 06018
www.vibranthealth.us
800-242-1835
	Lifetime
	Life's Basics
	Plant Protein
	(Pea, Hemp, Rice with Chia
	seed)
	Ingredients
	Pea Protein Isolate, Hemp
	Protein powder, Rice Protein
	Concentrate, Natural Vanilla
	Flavor, Fructose, Xylitol, Stevia
	and Salt.
	Serving size 35.1 g. (1
	        scoops, or 1 ounce)
	Protein 22 g 44%
	Formulated and distributed by:
	Life Time Nutritional
	Specialties, Inc
	Orange, CA 92865
	www.lifetimevitamins.com

The Ultimate Meal Ingredients organic Amaranth, millet, brown rice protein (75% concentrate), flax seed, spirulina … …others Serving size 40 g. (1 scoop) Protein 16 g The Ultimate Life Santa Barbara, CA 93140 www.ultimatelife.com	**Paradise** **Protein Greens** Pea protein isolate (non GMO) Serving Size 30.25 g (approx 2 scoops) Protein 22 grams Paradise Herbs, Inc. Huntington Beach, CA 92648 www.paradiseherbs.com
Peaceful Planet **The Supreme Meal** **Quinoa, Millet, & Amaranth** Ingredients Non-GMO protein blend: pea protein isolate, spirulina, rice protein concentrate, freeze-dried sprout blend (quinoa, milla, amaranth, broccoli), flax meal, … Serving size 35 g. Protein 17 g 34% Nutraceutical Corp. For Veg Life a Solaray brand Park City, Utah, 84060 www.nutraceuticalcom	**Raw Power!** Original protein superfood Ingredients organic Hemp protein powder (seed), brazil nut protein powder, maca powder (root), goji berry powder, mesquite powder (pod), meca powder (root extract). Serving size 28 g. (2 scoops,1oz.) Protein 8 g 16% Bazler Enterprises Coeur de Aleme, ID 83816 www.bazlerenterprises.com **Raw Power!** Green protein Superfood **With Barley grass powder** **Raw Power!** Chocolate flavor **Raw Power!** Vanilla
Biochem **Vegan Protein** Ingredients organic Pea Protein, Organic Hemp Seed Protein, Cranberry Protein, organic cane juice …others Serving size 36.5 g. (2 scoops) Protein 20 g 40% Biochem Hauppauge, NY 11788 www.biochem-fitness.com	**Plant Fusion - Vanilla Bean** Ingredients Amino Acid infused protein blend: Pea Protein Isolate, Artichoke Protein, Organic Sprouted Amaranth Powder and Organic Sprouted Quinoa Powder. Serving size 30 g. Protein 21 g. 42% www.plantfusion.net

Hemp - Maca Protein Powders

Ruth's Hemp and Flax Protein Powder 40% raw vegetarian protein Ingredients Certified Organic Hemp powder, certified organic sprouted, dehydrated flax. Serving size 30 g. Protein 12 g 18% **Ruth's Hemp Protein Power** Ingredients Certified Organic Hemp powder 50% raw vegetarian protein Serving size 30 g. Protein 15 g 23% Ruth's Hemp Foods, Inc. Toronto, Ontario, M5S 2S6 www.ruthshempfoods.com product of Canada	**Living Harvest Conscious Nutrition 100% Organic Hemp Protein** Organic; raw; cold processed; vegan; non-GMO; kosher; gluten free; Soy free; dairy free Ingredients Certified Organic Hemp Seed Serving size 30 g. Protein 14 g 30% Living Harvest Conscious Nutrition, Inc. www.livingharvest.com Product of Canada Living Harvest Conscious Nutrition, Inc. P.O. Box 4407 Portland, Oregon 97208 1-888-690-3958
Trader Joe's Organic Hemp Protein Powder Vanilla flavored Ingredients all organic Organic Hemp Protein, evaporated cane juice, vanilla Serving size 30 g. Protein 9 g 18% Trader Joe's Monrovia, CA 91016 Product of Canada	**Manitoba Harvest Hemp Protein Vanilla** Ingredients Organic Hemp protein powder, organic fair trade evaporated cane juice, organic vanilla flavor. Serving size 30 g. (4 Tbsp) Protein 11 g Manitoba Harvest Hemp Foods & Oils Winnipeg, Manitoba, Canada www.manitobaharvest.

Soy Protein Powders

Shaklee **Energizing Soy Protein** **Natural Vanilla** Non-GMO Soy Protein Ingredients Soy Lecithin, natural vanilla flavor, guar gum Serving size 28 g. Protein 14 g 28% Shaklee Corporation Pleasanton, CA 94588	**Peaceful Planet** **Super Spirulina Protein Shake** **French vanilla** Ingredients Non-GMO soy protein isolate, lecithin … blend…. Serving size 30.5 g. Protein 25 g 50% Nutraceutical Corp. www.nutracorp.com
Nature's Life **Organic Green Pro-96** **Soy Protein Powder** USDA Organic Ingredients: Organic Soy Protein (not genetically engineered), Phytogreen Blend (Oranic Spirulina, Organic Barley Grass, Chlorophyll and Organic Kelp) Serving size 25 g. Protein 17 g 34% **Nature's Life** **Organic Green Pro-96** Ingredients: Identity preserved (not genetically engineered) soy protein isolate, , Phytoblue Blend and more…… Serving size 31 g. Protein 25 g 50% www.natureslife.com Mfd. For Nature's Life Larkspur, CA 94939 800-247-6997	**Jarrow Formulas** **Iso-rich SOY** Ingredients Soy protein isolate (Non-GMO) and natural vanilla flavor. Serving size 29 g. Protein 25 g **Jarrow Formulas** **Fermented Soy Essence** Ingredients Organic soy milk yogurt (fermented with L. acidophilus, …) … lecithin (non-GMO) …. Serving size 28.5 g. Protein 11 g Jarrow Formulas Los Angeles, CA 90035 www.Jarrow.com

Rice Protein Powders

Amazing Grass **Amazing Meal, greens, protein,** **fruits and vegetables** **Original blend** Ingredients Organic rice protein, organic hemp protein, greens, blend.... Serving size 27 g. Protein 10 g 20% Amazing Grass San Francisco, CA 94147 www.amazinggrass.com	**Jarrow Formulas** **Brown Rice Protein** **Concentrate** **Non GMO vanilla** Ingredients organic Non-GMO brown rice protein, natural vanilla flavor, ... Serving size 15 g. (1 Tbsp) Protein 11 g Jarrow Formulas Los Angeles, CA 90035 www.Jarrow.com
NutriBiotic **Rice Protein** **Vanilla** Ingredients Enzymatically-processed rice protein from whole grain brown rice, natural vanilla flavor Serving size 15 g. (1 Tbsp) Protein 12 g NutriBiotic Lakeport, CA 95453 Nutribiotic.com	**Metagenics** **Ultra Meal Rice** **Natural Vanilla** Ingredients Rice protein concentrate, rice syrup solids, fructose, natural flavors,... Serving size 2 scoops (52 g.) Protein 15 g Metagenics 100 Avenida La Pata San Clemente, CA 92673 www.metagenics.com

Nature's Plus
Spiru-tein
High protein energy meal
Ingredients
Non-GMO soy protein blend
(rice, pea, soy,) fructose, ...
Serving size   34 g.
Protein   14 g 28%
Natural Organics Laboratories,
Inc.
Makers of Nature's Plus
Amityville, New York 11701
www.naturesplus.com
	Alive!
	Rice and Pea Protein
	Whole Food Energizer
	    Ultra Shake
	Vanilla flavor
	Ingredients
	Rice Protein and pea protein and
	blend....
	Serving size 39 g.
	Protein
	  Rice protein 7 g
	  Pea protein 6 g
	Nature's Way Products, Inc.
	Springville, Utah 84663
	www.naturesway.com

Notice:
        If this book is a significant help to your health or illness or degenerative disease, or even beneficial or a conversion or faith walk, please let us know. Myself and my associates are collecting testimonials and case studies for future works and possible a book. We are always interested when this book helps you in you're: body, soul or spirit. I do not always reply to email, but I always reply to a snail mail, drop me a letter.
        For other related books or activities see the website: www.jimtibbetts.com   Thank you and God bless.
            Sincerely in Christ
            Jim Tibbetts

Jim Tibbetts
P.O. Box 2533
Glenville, NY 12325
www.jimtibbetts.com

X. Appendix

A. Bio

James C. Tibbetts

Jim Tibbetts has an MBA (2009, Salve Regina, R.I.); an STL (1995) in Marian Studies (International Marian Research Institute, Univ. Dayton, Ohio) and an MA (1983) in theology (Univ. Steubenville, Ohio) and a BA (1976) in psychology, (Univ. of Buffalo, Buffalo, New York).

He is a member of Secular Franciscan Order (SFO), the K of C, the American Mariological Society and he is a Catholic charismatic, and a believer in Christian community.

James as a businessman ran various businesses. As a residential counselor Jim has worked with people with mental disabilities and mentally retardation in Maine and New York.

As a Catholic theologian and health advocate Jim has given talks at national conferences, Society meetings and given retreats on; Spirituality, Marian topics; on plant-based diets, fasting, healing and Christian meditation.

He has been into plant-based diets since about 1974, vegan and raw since 2001 and has done over 40 long juice fasts. He has studied yoga and Pilates and leads a Rosary yoga group.

Jim produced several DVD's on spiritual topics and mime. Jim is a professional mime (1978 to 2016); solo, duet and was a founding member (1991 to 2001) of the group "Christsong" on the life of Christ, which performed around the U.S., twice-toured England and appeared on television shows. "Tibbetts has studied his art under technique-oriented Marcel Marceau and personality-oriented Tony Montanaro. The result has been a critically acclaimed combination of the two." (*Arts & Entertainment*, Evening Express, Portland, ME.)

Jim has written journal and popular articles and has written over 20 books including:

1. Juice Fasting Simplified, a Practical Approach
2. A Diary on Juice Fasting
3. Living Green with Smoothies and the Culture of Life
4. Starving Cancer to Death, Nutritional Integrative Cancer Therapies, with Joseph Spaziani, MD
5. Starving into Remission: Alzheimer's, Parkinson's and Multiple Sclerosis - Nutritional Therapies
6. The Sower's Seeds of Remission and Curing: Alzheimer's, Parkinson's and MS! A Nutrition Therapy Novel
7. Superior Health for Astronauts as Raw Vegans A Nutrition Novel
8. The Bioethics of Drug Intervention
9. Christian Meditation, the Jesus Prayer and Praise
10. Jesus and Mary were Kosher Vegetarian, the Evidence from the Bible, the Early Church and Nutrition
11. Biblical Nutrition and Fasting
12. Biblical Nutrition; Forty Days of Meditations
13. Biblical Nutrition the Kosher Vegetarianism of Jesus and Judaism
14. Biblical Fasting
15. A Biblical Ballad of Mary Mother of Jesus
16. Biblical Titles of the Virgin Mary - 30 Day Meditation
17. Mary the Kosher Vegetarian, Impacting Climate Change
18. The Virgin Mary His Ark of the Covenant with Fr. Bill McCarthy
19. Christian Meditation Ancient and Modern, Eastern and Western with Fr. Bill McCarthy
20. Guadalupe the Tilma's Conquest - a historical novel
21. Q & A about Vegetarians and Health

For pictures see website: www.jimtibbetts.com

B. Endnotes

[1] Handel, Jacob, "Chlorophyll Supporter of all Human and Animal Life",
p. 32, 33, 56.

[2] Saunders, C. 1926. The nutritional value of chlorophyll as related to
hemoglobin formation. Proceedings of the Society for Experimental
Biology and Medicine (3172), p. 788-789: Cited in, ibid. Handel, Jacob,
"Chlorophyll Supporter...". p. 33.

[3] Smith, L. 1944. Chlorophyll: an experimental study of its water-soluble
derivatives. Remarks on the history, chemistry, toxicity and anti-bacterial
properties of water soluble chlorophyll derivatives as therapeutic agents.
American Journal of the Medical Sciences 207:647-654. Cited in, ibid.
Handel, Jacob, "Chlorophyll Supporter...". p. 33.

[4] Rothemund, P., McNary, R., and Inman, O. 1934. Occurrence of
decomposition products of chlorophyll II. Decomposition products of
chlorophyll in the stomach walls of herbivorous animals. *Journal of the
American Chemical Society* 56:2400-2403. Cited in, ibid. Handel, Jacob,
"Chlorophyll Supporter...". p. 33.

[5] Wigmore, Ann; Pattinson, Lee, *The Blending Book Maximizing
Nature's Nutrients*, (Avery, New York, N.Y., 1997 edition), p. 1.

[6] Wigmore, Ann; Pattinson, Lee, *The Blending Book,* p. 7.

[7] Wigmore, Ann; Pattinson, Lee, *The Blending Book,* p. 9.

[8] Wigmore, Ann; Pattinson, Lee, *The Blending Book,* p. 11.

[9] Wigmore, Ann; Pattinson, Lee, *The Blending Book,* p. 121.

[10] Boutenko, Victoria, *Green for Life*, (Raw Family Pub., 2005), p. 95.

[11] Boutenko, Victoria, *Green for Life*, (Raw Family Pub., 2005), p. 38.

[12] Gurskin, B. "Chlorophyll - Its Therapeutic Place in Acute and
Supporative Disease," *American Journal of Surgery* 49 (1940): 49-55.

[13] Levin, Buck, *Environmental Nutrition...*, p. 179, citing: Murphy R. and
Harvey C. (1985). Residues and metabolites of selected persistent
halogenated hydrocarbons in blood from a general population survey.
Environ Health Perspect 60:115-120.

[14] Ibid., p. 179, citing: Lordo RA, Dinh KT, and Schwemberger JG.
(1996). Semivolatile organic compounds in adipose tissue: estimated
averages for the US population and selected subpopulations. *Am J Pub
Heal* 86(9):1253-1259.

[15] Ibid., p. 215, citing: Stehr-Green PA. (1989). Demographic and
seasonal influences on human serum pesticide residue levels. J *Toxicol
Environ Heal* 27(4):405-421.

[16] Ibid., p. 181, citing: Henriksen GL, Ketchum NS, Michalek JE it al.
(1997). Serum dioxin and diabetes mellitus in veterans of Operation
Ranch Hand. *Epidem* 8(3):252-258.

[17] Ibid., p. 181, citing: Hill RH Jr, Ashley DL, Head Sl et al. (1995). P-
dichlorobenzene exposure among 1,000 adults in the United States. *Arch*

Environ Health 50(4):277-280.

[18] Ibid., p. 181, citing: Hammand TA, Sexton M, and Langenberg P. (1996). Relationship between blood lead and dietary iron intake in preschool children. *Ann Epidemiol* 6(1):30-33. Also: Kim R, Landrigan c, Mossmann P et al. (1997). Age and secular trends in bone lead levels in middle-aged and elderly men: three-year longitudinal follow-up in the Normative Aging Study. *Am J Epidemiol* 146(7):586-591.

[19] Ibid., Levin, Buck, *Environmental Nutrition,* p. 181, citing: Yamamura Y, Yoshinaga Y, Arai F et al. (1994). Background levels of total mercury concentrations in blood and urine. *Sangyo Igaku* 36(2):66-69.

[20] Ibid., Levin, Buck, *Environmental Nutrition,* p. 181, citing: Chia SE, chan OY, Sam CT et al. (1994). Blood cadmium levels in nonoccupationally exposed adult subjects in Singapore. *Sci Total Environ* 145(1-2):119-123.

[21] Ibid., Levin, Buck, *Environmental Nutrition,* p. 181, citing: Wolff MS, Anderson HA, and selikoff IJ. (1982). Human tissue burdens of halogenated aromatic chemicals in Michigan. *JAMA* 247(15):2112-2116.

[22] Ibid., Levin, Buck, *Environmental Nutrition,* p. 181, citing: Hill RH Jr, Head SL, Baker S et al. (1995). Pesticide residues in urine of adults living in the United States: reference range concentrations. *Environ Res* 71(2):99-108.

[23] Ibid., p. 215, citing: Guengerich FP and Shimada T, *op. cit.*

[24] Ibid., Levin, Buck, *Environmental Nutrition,* p. 215, citing: Nakajima T and Wang RS. (1994). Induction of cytochrome P450 by toluene. Int J Biochem 26(12):133301340.

[25] Ibid., p. 215, citing: Ungv-rg G. (1990). The effect of xylene exposure on the liver. *Acta Morphol Hungar* 38:245-258.

[26] Ibid., Levin, Buck, *Environmental Nutrition,* p. 215, citing: Casazza JP, Felver ME, and Veech RL. (1984). The metabolism of acetone in the rat. *J Biol Chem* 259:231-236.

[27] Ibid., Levin, Buck, *Environmental Nutrition,* p. 215, citing: Albores A, Sinal CJ, Cherian MG et al. (1995). Selective increase of rat lung cytochrome P450 1A1 dependent monooxygenase activity after acute sodium arsenite administration. *Can J Physiol Pharmocol* 73(1):153-158.

[28] Ibid., Levin, Buck, *Environmental Nutrition,* p. 215, citing: Keyon EM, Kraichely RE, Hudson KT, it al. (1996). Differences in rates of benzene metabolism correlate with observed genotoxicity. *Toxicol Appl Pharmacol* 136(1): 49-56.

[29] Ibid., Levin, Buck, *Environmental Nutrition,* p. 215, citing: Zheng J and Hanzlik RP. (1992). Bromo(monohydroxyl)phenyl mercapturic acids: a new class of merapturic acids from bromobenzene-treated rats. *Drug Metabol Dispos* 20:688-694.

[30] Ibid., Levin, Buck, *Environmental Nutrition,* p. 215, citing: Guengerich FP and Shimada T. (1992). Human cytochrome P450 enzymes and chemical carcinogenesis. Chapter 2. In: Jeffrey EH. (Ed). Human drug metabolism from molecular biology to man. *CRC Press,*

Boca Raton, pp. 5-12.

[31] Ibid., Levin, Buck, *Environmental Nutrition,* p. 215, citing: Guengerich FP. (1994). Metabolism and genotoxicity of dihaloalkanes. *Adv Pharmacol* 27:211-236.

[32] Ibid., Levin, Buck, *Environmental Nutrition,* p. 215, citing: Cheever KL, Cholkis JM, et-Hawari AM et al. (1990). Ethlyene dichloride: the influence of disulfiram or ethanol on oncogenicity, metabolism and DNA covalent binding in rats. *Fund Appl Toxicol* 14(2):243-261.

[33] Ibid., Levin, Buck, *Environmental Nutrition,* p. 215, citing: Lapadula DM. (1991). Induction of cytochrome P450 isozymes by simultaneous inhalation exposure of hens to n-hexane and methyl iso-butyl ketone (MiBK). *Biochem Pharmacol* 41(6-7):877-883.

[34] Ibid., Levin, Buck, *Environmental Nutrition,* p. 215, citing: Kocarek TA. (1991). Selective induction of cytochrome P450e by kepone (chlordecone) in primary clutures of adult rat hepatocytes, *Mol Pharmacol* 40(2):203-210.

[35] Ibid., Levin, Buck, *Environmental Nutrition,* p. 215, citing: Stresser DM and Kupfer D. (1997). Catalytic characteristics of CYP3A4: requirement for a phenolic fuction in ortho hydroxylation of estradiol and mono-O-demethylated methoxychlor. *Biochem* 36(8):2203-2210.

[36] Ibid., Levin, Buck, *Environmental Nutrition,* p. 215, citing: Vezina M, Kobusch AB, du Souich P et al. (1990). Potentiation of chloroform induced hepatotoxicity by metyl isobuty ketone and two metabolites. *Can J Physiol Pharmacol* 68(8):1055-1061.

[37] Ibid., Levin, Buck, *Environmental Nutrition,* p. 215, citing: Hogan GK, Smith RG, and Cornish HH. (1976). Studies on the microsomal conversion of dichloromethane to carbon monoxide. *Toxicol App Pharmacol* 37:112-119.

[38] Ibid., Levin, Buck, *Environmental Nutrition,* p. 214, citing: Levin W et al. (1982). Oxidative metabolism of polycyclic aromatic hydrocarbons to ultimate carcinogens. *Drug Metab Rev* 13:555-580.

[39] Winter, *Poisons in Your Food,* p. 5, citing: Howard J. Sanders, "Food Additives," *Chemical and Engineering News,* October 17, 1966. James L. Goddard, M.S., FDA Commissioner, tape-recorded interview with author, May, 1968.

[40] Winter, *Poisons in Your Food,* p. 5, citing: Pharmaceutical Manufacturers Association, Washington, D.C., fact booklet, 1967.

[41] Cousens, Gabriel, M.D., *Rainbow Green Live-Food Cuisine,* p. xiv.

[42] Airola, Paavo, N.D., PhD., *Juice Fasting,* (Health Publishers, Phoenix, Arizona), 1971, p. 40.

[43] Airola, Paavo, N.D., PhD., *Juice Fasting,* p. 39, 40, 38.

[44] Openshaw, Robyn, *The Green Smoothies Diet, the Natural Program for Extraordinary Health,* (Ulysses Press, Berkeley, CA, 2009). www.ulyssespress.com

[45] Her website: GreenSmoothiesGirl.com was the place she did the survey for the study.

[46] Openshaw, Robyn, *The Green Smoothies Diet,* p. 56-59.

[47] Cement, Brian, *Living Foods for Optimum Health,* (Prima Publishing, Hppocrates Health Institute, FL, 1996).

[48] Gurskin, B. "Chlorophyll - Its Therapeutic Place in Acute and Supporative Disease," *American Journal of Surgery* 49 (1940): 49-55.

[49] Miller, Lois, M. "The Green Magic of Chlorophyll," *Reader's Digest* (April, 1941): 30-32.

[50] John Gainer, "Now the Villain is Protein," *Science News* (August 21, 1971): 123-24.

[51] Meyerowitz, Steve, *Wheatgrass Nature's Finest Medicine,* (Book Publishing Company, TN), 1999.

[52] Ann Wigmore, *Be Your Own doctor* (Garden City Park, NY: Avery Publishing Group, 1982).

[53] Walters, Richard, *Options the Alternative Cancer Therapy Book,* Avery Pub. Group, Inc., 1992, p. 147.

[54] Ibid., Walters, p. 148.

[55] Boutenko, Victoria, *Green for Life,* (Raw Family Pub., 2005), p. 110.

[56] Walters, Richard, Options the Alternative Cancer Therapy Book, p.151 citing: Kistine Nolfi, M.D., *My Experience With Living Foods: The Raw Food Treatment of Cancer and Other Diseases* (Mokelumne Hill, CA: Health Research), p. 14.

[57] Cousens, Gabriel, *Conscious Eating,* p. 587-8.

[58] Kulvinskas, *Survival Into...,* p. 27. Citing: (a) Annand, J.c., L. Coll. *Gen. Pract.,* 2:365, 1959. (b) Yarushalmy T. Hilleboe, H.E., N.Y. State *T. Med.* 53:2343, 1957.

[59] Ibid., Kulvinskas, Survival Into..., p. 27. Citing: (a) Oliver M.F., *Lancet,* 1:653, 1962. (b) McDonald L., Edgill M. *Lancet,* 1:996; 1958.

[60] Kulvinskas, *Survival into the 21st Century,* p. 53, citing: Paloscia; Pollotten; "Chlorophyl Therapy" Lotta. *Contra. Tuberc.* 22: 738, 1952.

[61] Kulvinskas, *Survival into the 21st Century,* p. 53, citing: "Results of Chlorophyl Therapy," Bull Assoc. Franc Poletude due *Cancer,* 24: 15, 1935.

[62] Kulvinskas, *Survival into the 21st Century,* p. 53, citing: Plagniel, "Remarkable Tonic Power of Chlorophyll Pigment in Asthenic Toxemia of Cancer," *J. de Med.* De Paris, 53: 664, 1933.

[63] Kulvinskas, *Survival into the 21st Century,* p. 53, citing: "Chlorophyll Therapy for Cancer," *Progress. Med.,* Ap. 6, 1935, p. 583.

[64] Meyerowitz, Steve, *Wheat Grass, Nature's Finest Medicine,* p. 70, citing: Dr. Mahnaz Badamchian of the Dept. of Biochemistry and Molecular Biology, George Washing Univ., Medical Center research: Anti-tumor properties of barley leaf extract (BLE) on human prostrate, breast and melanoma cancer.

[65] Meyerowitz, Steve, *Wheat Grass, Nature's Finest Medicine,* p. 69, citing: Inhibition of In Vitro Metabolic Activation of Carcinogens by Wehat Sprout Extracts, By Chiu-Nan Lai, B Dabney, C. Shaw, Dept of Biology, Unive of Texas System Cancer Center, M.D. Anderson Hospital

and Tumor institute, Houston, TX. *Nutrition and Cancer* . Vol. 1, no. 1.
P-27-30. Fall, 1978.

[66] Kulvinskas, *Survival into the 21st Century*, p. 54, citing: Smith,
"Remarks Upon the History, Chemistry, Toxicity and Antibacterial
Properties of Watersoluble Chlorophyll Derivatives as Therapeutic
Agents," *Am. J. Med. Soc.* 207:649, 1944.

[67] Kulvinskas, *Survival into the 21st Century*, p. 54, citing: Bowers W.S.,
"Chlorophyl in Wound Healing and Suppurative Disease",
Am. J. Surg. 73, 1947.

[68] Kulvinskas, *Survival into the 21st Century*, p. 54, citing: Rafsky,
Krieger, "Treatment of Intestinal Diseases with Solutions of Water
Soluble Chlorophyl," *Rev. Gastroentology*, 15: 549, 1948.

[69] Day, Lorraine, MD, *Getting Started...*, p. 161, citing: *Environmental
Nutrition*, 1994, 3; *The American Journal of Clinical Nutrition*,
1990;51:656-657.

[70] Siebold, in *Cereal Grass: Nature's Greatest Health Gift*.

[71] Siebold, Ronald, M.S., *Cereal Grass: Nature's Greatest Health Gift*
(NTC/Contemporary Pub., 1991).

[72] Dubin, Reese, *Miracle Food Cures from the Bible*, (Prentice Hall,
Paramus, NJ) 1999, p. 130.

[73] Siebold, in *Cereal Grass: Nature's Greatest Health Gift*.

[74] Siebold, in *Cereal Grass: Nature's Greatest Health Gift*.

[75] Siebold, in *Cereal Grass: Nature's Greatest Health Gift*.

[76] Dubin, Reese, *Miracle Food Cures from the Bible*, p. 129.

[77] Dubin, Reese, *Miracle Food Cures from the Bible*, p. 132.

[78] Dubin, Reese, *Miracle Food Cures from the Bible*, p. 133.

[79] Dubin, Reese, *Miracle Food Cures from the Bible*, p. 133.

[80] *Chlorophyllin Reduces Aflatoxin Indicators Among People At High
Risk for Liver Cancer*. Johns Hopkins University Bloomberg School of
Public Health, Baltimore, MD. Proceedings of the National Academy of
Sciences. November 27, 2001. Cited by Boutenko, Victoria, *Green for
Life*, p. 94.

[81] Chernomorsky, S. et al. "Effect of Dietary Chlorophyll Derivatives on
Mutagenesis and Tumor Cell Growth." *Teratogenesis Carcinogenesis*,
79:313-322, 1999. Cited by Boutenko, *Green for Life*, p. 95.

[82] Vlad M. et al. *Effect of Cuprofilin on Experimental Atherosclerosis*.
Romania: Institute of Public Health and Medical Research, University of
Medicine and Pharmacy, Cluj-Napoca, 1995. Cited by Boutenko,
Victoria, *Green for Life*, p. 95.

[83] Handel, Jacob, "Chlorophyll Supporter of all Human and Animal
Life", *Healing Our World*, (Hippocrates Health Institute, 2010, Vol. 30,
Issue 3), p. 32, 33, 56.

[84] Carpenter, E. 1949. Clinical experiences with chlorophyll preparations
with a particular reference to chronic osteomyelitis and chronic ulcers.
American Journal of Surgery. Feb. 1949: Cited in, ibid. Handel, Jacob,
"Chlorophyll Supporter...". p. 32.

[85] Saunders, C. 1926. The nutritional value of chlorophyll as related to hemoglobin formation. Proceedings of the Society for Experimental Biology and Medicine (3172), p. 788-789: Cited in, ibid. Handel, Jacob, "Chlorophyll Supporter...". p. 32.

[86] Lai, C., Butler, M., and Matney, T. 1980. Antimutagenic activities of common vegetables and their chlorophyll content. *Mutation Research* 77:245-250. Cited in, ibid. Handel, Jacob, "Chlorophyll Supporter...", p. 32.

[87] Spector, H. and Calloway, D. 1959. Reduction of x-radiation mortality by cabbage and broccoli. Proceedings of the Society for Experimental Biology and Medicine 100:405-407. Cited in, ibid. Handel, Jacob, "Chlorophyll Supporter...", p. 32.

[88] Calloway, D., Newell, G., Calhoun, W. and Munson, A. 1962. Further studies of the influence on diet on radiosensitivity of guinea pigs, with special reference to broccoli and alfalfa. *Journal of Nutrition* 79:340-348. Cited in, ibid. Handel, Jacob, "Chlorophyll Supporter...". p. 32.

[89] Smith, L. 1944. Chlorophyll: an experimental study of its water-soluble derivatives. Remarks on the history, chemistry, toxicity and anti-bacterial properties of water soluble chlorophyll derivatives as therapeutic agents. *American Journal of the Medical Sciences* 207:647-654. Cited in, ibid. Handel, Jacob, "Chlorophyll Supporter...". p. 32.

[90] Offenkrantz, W. 1950. Water-soluble chlorophyll in the treatment of peptic ulcers of long duration. *Review of Gastroenterology* 17:359-367. Cited in, ibid. Handel, Jacob, "Chlorophyll Supporter...". p. 32.

[91] Ohtake, H., Nonaka, S., Sawada, Y., Hagiwara, Y., Hagiwara, H., and Kubota, K. 1985. Studies on the constituents of green juice from young barley leaves. Effect on dietarily induced hypercholesterolemia in rats. *Journal of the Pharmaceutical Society of Japan* 105:1052-71. Calloway, D., Newell, G., Calhoun, W. and Munson, A. 1962. Further studies of the influence on diet on radiosensitivity of guinea pigs, with special reference to broccoli and alfalfa. *Journal of Nutrition* 79:340-348. Cited in, ibid. Handel, Jacob, "Chlorophyll Supporter...". p. 32.

[92] Smith, L. 1944. Chlorophyll: an experimental study of its water-soluble derivatives. Remarks on the history, chemistry, toxicity and anti-bacterial properties of water soluble chlorophyll derivatives as therapeutic agents. *American Journal of the Medical Sciences* 207:647-654. Cited in, ibid. Handel, Jacob, "Chlorophyll Supporter...". p. 32.

[93] Carpenter, E. 1949. Clinical experiences with chlorophyll preparations with a particular reference to chronic osteomyelitis and chronic ulcers. *American Journal of Surgery*. Feb. 1949: Cited in, ibid. Handel, Jacob, "Chlorophyll Supporter...". p. 33.

[94] Saunders, C. 1926. The nutritional value of chlorophyll as related to hemoglobin formation. Proceedings of the Society for Experimental Biology and Medicine (3172), p. 788-789: Cited in, ibid. Handel, Jacob, "Chlorophyll Supporter...". p. 33.

[95] Smith, L. 1944. Chlorophyll: an experimental study of its water-

soluble derivatives. Remarks on the history, chemistry, toxicity and anti-bacterial properties of water soluble chlorophyll derivatives as therapeutic agents. *American Journal of the Medical Sciences* 207:647-654. Cited in, ibid. Handel, Jacob, "Chlorophyll Supporter...". p. 33.

[96] Rothemund, P., McNary, R., and Inman, O. 1934. Occurrence of decomposition products of chlorophyll.II. Decomposition products of chlorophyll in the stomach walls of herbivorous animals. *Journal of the American Chemical Society* 56:2400-2403. Cited in, ibid. Handel, Jacob, "Chlorophyll Supporter...". p. 33.

[97] Hughes, J. and Latner, A. 1936. Chlorophyll and haemoglobin regeneration after haemorrhage, *Journal of Physiology* 86:388-395. Cited in, ibid. Handel, Jacob, "Chlorophyll Supporter...". p. 33.

[98] Patek, A. 1936. Chlorophyll and regeneration of the blood. *Archives of Internal Medicine* 57:73-84. Cited in, ibid. Handel, Jacob, "Chlorophyll Supporter...". p. 33.

[99] Scott, E. and Delor, C. 1933. Nutritional anemia. *Ohio State Medical Journal* 29:165-169. Cited in, ibid. Handel, Jacob, "Chlorophyll Supporter...". p. 32.

[100] Hammel-Dupont, C. and Bessman, S. 1970. The stimulation of hemoglobin synthesis by porphyrins. *Biochemical Medicine* 4:55-60. Cited in, ibid. Handel, Jacob, "Chlorophyll Supporter...". p. 33.

[101] Handel, Jacob, "Chlorophyll Supporter of all Human and Animal Life", p. 32, 33, 56.

[102] Saunders, C. 1926. The nutritional value of chlorophyll as related to hemoglobin formation. Proceedings of the Society for Experimental Biology and Medicine (3172), p. 788-789: Cited in, ibid. Handel, Jacob, "Chlorophyll Supporter...". p. 33.

[103] Kimm, S., Tschai, B., and Park, S. 1982. Antimutagenic activity of chlorophyll to direct and indirect-acting mutagens and its contents in the vegetables. *Korean Journal of Biochemistry* 14:1-7. Saunders, C. 1926. The nutritional value of chlorophyll as related to hemoglobin formation. Proceedings of the Society for Experimental Biology and Medicine (3172), p. 788-789: Cited in, ibid. Handel, Jacob, "Chlorophyll Supporter...". p. 33.

[104] Ong, T., Whong, W., Stewart, J. and Brockman, H. 1986. Chlorophyllin: a potent antimutagen against environmental and dietary complex mixtures. *Mutation Research* 173:111-15. Saunders, C. 1926. The nutritional value of chlorophyll as related to hemoglobin formation. Proceedings of the Society for Experimental Biology and Medicine (3172), p. 788-789: Cited in, ibid. Handel, Jacob, "Chlorophyll Supporter...", p. 33.

[105] Spector, H. and Calloway, D. 1959. Reduction of x-radiation mortality by cabbage and broccoli. Proceedings of the Society for Experimental Biology and Medicine 100:405-407. Cited in, ibid. Handel, Jacob, "Chlorophyll Supporter...", p. 56.

[106] Calloway, D., Newell, G., Calhoun, W. and Munson, A. 1962.

Further studies of the influence on diet on radiosensitivity of guinea pigs, with special reference to broccoli and alfalfa. *Journal of Nutrition* 79:340-348. Cited in, ibid. Handel, Jacob, "Chlorophyll Supporter...". p. 56.

[107] Handel, Jacob, "Chlorophyll Supporter of all Human and Animal Life", p. 32, 33, 56.

[108] Timon, Mark, "What are Green Foods?" (December 2009) Vibrant Health website.

[109] Joseph, James, Ph.D.; Nadeau, Daniel, M.D.; Underwood, Anne, *The Color Code a Revolutionary Eating Plan for Optimum Health*, (Hyperion, New York, NY), 2002, p. 3.

[110] Joseph, James, Ph.D.; Nadeau, Daniel, M.D.; Underwood, Anne, *The Color Code a Revolutionary Eating Plan for Optimum Health*, (Hyperion, New York, NY), 2002, p. 11.

[111] Joseph, Nadeau, Underwood, *The Color Code*, p. 8.

[112] Joseph, Nadeau, Underwood, *The Color Code*, p. 9.

[113] Joseph, Nadeau, Underwood, *The Color Code*, p. 14.

[114] Joseph, Nadeau, Underwood, *The Color Code*, p. 15.

[115] Joseph, Nadeau, Underwood, *The Color Code*, p. 16.

[116] Joseph, Nadeau, Underwood, *The Color Code*, p. 26.

[117] Jensen Bernard, D.C., PhD. *Tissue Cleansing Through Bowel Management*, Escondido, CA: Bernard Jensen Publishing, 1981. Cited in Boutenko, Victoria, *Green for Life*, p. 48.

[118] Mosseri, Albert. Le Jeune, Meilleur. *Remede de la Nature*. France: Aquarius, 1993. Cited in Boutenko, Victoria, *Green for Life*, p. 53.

[119] Boutenko, Victoria, *Green for Life*, p. 53.

[120] American Heart Association, 2004. Accessible at: www.americanheart.org: Cited in Boutenko, Victoria, *Green for Life*, (Raw Family Publishing, OR), p. 53.

[121] Boutenko, Victoria, *Green for Life*, p. 54.

[122] Boutenko, Victoria, *Green for Life*, p. 59.

[123] Walker WA. Isselbacher KJ. "Uptake and transport of macromolecules by the intestine. Possible role in clinical disorders." *Gastroenterology*: 67:531-50, 1974. Cited in Boutenko, Victoria, *Green for Life*, p. 47.

[124] Campbell, T. Colin, Ph.D. *The China Study*. (Texas: Benbella Books 2004).

[125] Boutenko, Victoria, *Green for Life*, p. 47.

[126] Cousens, Gabriel, MD, *Rainbow Green Live-Food Cuisine*, North Atlantic Books, Berkeley, CA., 2003, pp. 19-23.

[127] Graham, Doug, *Grain Damage* (Storrington, W. Sussex, 1998, Rozalind Gruben).

[128] Wolfe, David, *The Sunfood Diet Success System, Eating for Beauty*, (Maul Bros. Pub., 2002).

[129] Boutenko, Victoria, *12 Steps to Raw Foods How to End Your Addiction to Cooked Foods*, Raw Family Publishing, Ashland, OR., 2002.

[130] Rhio, *Hooked on Raw, Rejuvenate your Body and Soul with Nature's Living Foods*, (Beso Entertainment, 2000).

[131] Sarno, Chad, *Vital Creations, An Organic Life Experience*, (www.rawchef.org, 2002).

[132] Juliano, *Raw the Uncook Book New Vegetarian Food for Life*, (Harper Collins Publishers, New York, N.Y., 1999).

[133] Shannon, Nomi, *The Raw Gourmet*, (Alive Books, Burnaby, BC, Canada, 1990).

[134] Baker, Elizabeth, The UnCook Book Raw Food Adventures to a New Health High, (ProMotion Publishing, San Diego, CA, 1996).

[135] Patenaude, Frederic, *The Sunfood Cuisine a Practical Guide to Raw Vegetarian Cuisine*, (San Diego, CA., 2001).

[136] Cobb, Brenda, *The Living Foods Lifestyle*, (Living Soul Publishing, Atlanta, GA, 2003).

[137] Trotter, Charlie; Klein, Roxanne, *RAW*, (Ten Speed Press, Berkley, CA., 2003).

[138] Shazzie, *Shazzie's Detox Delights*, (Rawcreation limited, 2001).

[139] Ferrara, Alex, *The Raw Food Primer*, (Council Oak Books, San Francisco, Tulsa, OK, 2003).

[140] Love, Elaine, *Elaine's Pure Joy Kitchen, Raw, Organic, Vegan, Recipes,* (www.purejoylivingfoods.com) 1998.

[141] Boutenko, Igor, *Igor's Live Flat Bread*, (Raw Family Publishing, 2005).

[142] Boutenko, Sergei; Boutenko, Valya, *Eating without Heating*, (Raw Family Publishing, 2004).

[143] Wandling, Julie, *Thank God for Raw*, (Healthy 4 Him Publishing, Akron, OH, 2002).

[144] Nison, Paul, *The Raw Life*, (343 Publishing Company, New York, N.Y., 2000).

[145] Arlin, Stephen, *Raw Power*, (Maul Brothers Publishing, San Diego, CA., 1998).

[146] Young, *Sick and Tired?*, Ibid.

[147] Clement, Brian, PhD., *Living Foods for Optimum Health*, (Prima Pub, Hippocrates Inst. FL, 1996).

[148] Clement, Anna Maria, PhD., *Healthful Cuisine*, (Healthful Communications, Juno Beach, FL, 2006).

[149] Soria, Cherie, *Angel Foods*, (Heartstar Productions, Santa Barbara, CA., 1996).

[150] Tibbetts, James, *Superior Health with a Living Foods Lifestyle*, (2003; www.jimtibbetts.com).

[151] Mars, Brigitte, *Rawsome! Maximizing Health, Energy and Culinary Delight with the Raw Foods Diet*, (Basic Health Publications, NJ, 2004).

[152] Levin, James, MD; Cederquist Natalie, *Vibrant Living*, (GLO, Inc., La Jolla, CA, 1993; 2001).

[153] Safron, Jeremy, A.; Underkoffler, Renee, *The Raw Truth the Art of Loving Foods*, (Loving Foods, Inc.,

Paia, HI, 1997).
[154] Romano, Rita, *Dining in the Raw Groundbreaking Natural Cuisine that Combines the Techniques of Macrobiotic, Vegan, Allergy-free, and Raw Food Disciplines*, (Kensigton Pub., 1992).
[155] Jubb, David & Annie Padden, *Life Food Recipe Book, Living on Life Force*, (North Atlantic Books, CA., 2003).
[156] Safron, Jeremy, *The Raw Truth, the Art of Preparing Living Foods*, (Celestial Arts, Berkeley, 2003).
[157] Markowitz, Elysa, *Warming Up to Living Foods*, (Book Publishing Company, 1998).
[158] Schnitzer, Johann, *Schnitzer-Intensive Nutrition, Schnitzer-Normal Nutrition*, (Schnitzer Publishers, Black Forest, W. Germany, 2002, tenth revised edition).
[159] Gerson, Charlotte, Walker, Morton, DPM, *The Gerson Therapy*, (Kensington Publishing Corp., New York, N.Y., 2001), p. 94, 98.
[160] Sheraton (Dina), Jameth, ND, Sheraton (Sproul), Kim, ND, *Uncooking with Jameth and Kim*, (Healthforce Publishing, 1991-2001).
[161] Malkmus, George H., *God's Way to Ultimate Health*, (Hallelujah Acres Pub, Shelby, NC, 1995).
[162] Malkmus, Rhonda, J., *Recipes for Life*, (Hallelujah Acres Pub., Shelby, NC, 2001).
[163] Diamond, Harvey & Marilyn, *Fit for Life II: Living Health*, (Warner Books, New York, NY, 1987).
[164] Smith, Melissa, D., *Going Against the Grain*, (Contemporary Books, New York), 2002.
[165] Horne, Ross, *Improving on Pritikin - You can do Better!*, (Happy Landings Pty Ltd, Australia, 1988),
p. 10. citing, Dr. Emmet Densmore and Dr. Charles De Lacy Evenas of England.
[166] Cobb, Brenda, *The Living Foods Lifestyle*, Living Soul Publishing, Atlanta, GA, 2003, p. 88.
[167] Cousens, Gabriel, *Conscious Eating*, p. 763.
[168] Cousens, Gabriel, *Conscious Eating*, p. 763.
[169] Cousens, Gabriel, MD. *Rainbow Green Live-Food Cuisine*, p. 19.
[170] Smith, Melissa Diane, *Going Against the Grain*, (Contemporary Books/McGraw-Hill, 2002), p. 47; citing: J. Saleron et al, "Dietary fiber, glycemic load, and the risk of non-insulin-dependent diabetes mellitus in women," *Journal of the American Medical Association* 277 (1997): 472-77.
[171] Smith, *Going Against the Grain*, citing: D.R. Jacobs, Jr. et al., "Whole-grain intake may reduce the risk of ischemic heart disease death in postmenopausal women: The Iowa Women's Health Study," *American Journal of Clinical Nutrition* 68 (1998): 248-57.
[172] Smith, *Going Against the Grain*, p 47.
[173] Nison, Paul, *Raw Knowledge II*, p. 223, citing a Dr. Vivian Ventrano interview.

[174] Meyerowitz, Steve, Sprouts the Miracle Food, the Complete Guide to Sprouting, (Sproutman Publications, P.O. Box 1100, Great Barrington, MA., 01230, www.sproutman.com; 2010).

[175] Baker, Elizabeth, *The Gourmet Uncook Book, The Elegance of Raw Foods*, Promotion Publishing, San Diego, CA., 1996, p. 23-24.

[176] Baroody, Theodore, N.D., D.C., Ph.D., Alkalize or Diet Superior Health Through Proper Alkaline-Acid Balance (Holographic Health Press, Waynesville, N.C.), 2001, p. 15, 22.

[177] Young, Robert, PhD., Sick and Tired, p. 63-64.

[178] Young, Robert, PhD., Sick and Tired, p. 51, 61.

[179] Aihara, *Acid and Alkaline*, p. 17.

[180] Rogers, Sherry, MD, Pain Free in 6 Weeks, Prestige Publishing, Syracuse, NY, 2001, p. 316.

[181] Aihara, Herman, *Acid and Alkaline*, (George Ohsawa Macrobiotic Foundation, Oroville, CA), 1986 (1971), p. 114.

[182] Pierce, Tanya Harter, *Outsmart your Cancer*, Thoughtworks Publishing, Nevada, 2004, p. 274, citing: www.gethealthyagain.com.

[183] Brewer, A. Keith, Ph.D., "The High pH Therapy for Cancer, Tests on Mice and Humans," *Pharmacology Biochemistry and Behavior*, vol. 21, suppl. 1, 1984, pp. 1-5.

[184] Brewer, Keith, Cancer: *The Mechanism Involved and a High pH Therapy, 1978 Papers of A.Keith Brewer, Ph.D., and coauthors.* A Keith Brewer Foundation, 325 N. Central Avenue, Richland Center, WI 53581.

[185] Sartori HE. Nutrients and cancer: an introduction to cesium therapy. *Pharmacol Biochem Behav.* 1984;1:7-10.

[186] Dr. Otto Warburg. K. Triltsch. The Prime Cause and Prevention of Cancer. 2d. rev edition (1969) 16 pages. Lecture delivered to Nobel Laureates on June 30, 1966 at Lindau, Lake Constance, Germany. English Edition by Dean Burk National Cancer Institute, Bethesda, Maryland, USA. Accessible at: http://www.mmfnd.org/NL/ONN/WS/ozon005.html. Cited in, Boutenko, Victoria, *Green for Life*, (Raw Family Publishing, 2005), p. 80-81.

[186] Boutenko, Victoria, *Green for Life*, (Raw Family Pub., 2005), p. 82.

[187] Boutenko, Victoria, *Green for Life*, (Raw Family Pub., 2005), p. 82.

[188] Boutenko, Victoria, *Green for Life*, (Raw Family Pub., 2005), p. 82.

[189] Boutenko, Victoria, *Green for Life*, p. 84-85.

[190] Wolverton, B.C., Dr., *How to Grow Fresh Air*, (Penguin Books, New York, 1996), chapter 1.

[191] Wolverton, *How to Grow Fresh Air*, chapter 2.

[192] Wolverton, *How to Grow Fresh Air*, chapter 3.

[193] Chisaka T, et al. The effect of crude drugs on experimental hypercholesteremia: mode of action of (1)-epigallocatechin gallate in tea leaves. *Chem Pharm Bull* (Tokyo). 1988;36:227-33.

[194] Fujita Y, et. Al. Inhibitory effect of (-)-epigallocatechin gallate on carcinogenesis with N-ethyl-N'-nitro-N-nitrosoguanidine in mouse duodenum. *Jpn J Cancer Res.* 1989;80:503-5.

[195]   Fujiki H, et al. New antitumor promoters: (-)-epigallocatechin gallate and sarcophytols A and B. *Basic Life Sci.* 1990;52:205-12.
[196]   Fujiki H. (-)-epigallocatechin gallate (EGCG), cancer preventive agent. Fourth Chemical Congress of North America. New York:American Chemical Society, 1991.
[197]   Yang C, et al. Protection against stomach, lung and esophageal carcinogenesis by green tea. Fourth Chemical Congress of North America. New York:American Chemical Society, 1991.
[198]   Cassileth, Complementary Therapies: the American Experience, p. 18.
[199]   Cassileth, Barrie R. Ph.D., *Complementary Therapies: the American Experience*, Support Care Cancer, (2000) 8:16-23. Integrative Medicine Service, Memorial Sloan-Kettering Cancer Center, New York, N.Y.
[200]   Baker, Sidney MacDonald, M.D., *Detoxification and Healing: The Key to Optimal Health,* Keats Publishing, New Canaan, CT., 1997, p. 157-158.
[201]   Hildenbrand, G., and S. Gavin. "Five-Year Survival Rates of Melanoma Patients Treated by Diet Therapy after the Manner of Gerson: A Retrospective Review." *Alternative Therapies in Health and Medicine* 1:4 (1995), 29-37.
[202]   Hildenbrand, Gar, J., *Natuopath Med.,* 1996; 6(1):49-56.
[203]   The Raw Family website 2009 or earlier.
[204]   The Raw Family website October 29, 2009 or earlier.
[205]   The Raw Family website 2009 or earlier.
[206]   Walker WA. Isselbacher KJ. "Uptake and transport of macromolecules by the intestine. Possible role in clinical disorders." *Gastroenterology*: 67:531-50, 1974. Cited in Boutenko, Victoria, *Green for Life*, p. 47.
[207]   Minocha Anil M.D., Carrol David. *Natural Stomach Care: Treating and Preventing Digestive Disorders with the Best of Eastern and Western Healing Therapies*. New York: Penguin Group, 2003. Cited in Boutenko, Victoria, *Green for Life*, p. 62.
[208]   Boutenko, Victoria, *Green for Life*, p. 62, citing: Elson M. Haas M.D. *Staying Healthy with Nutrition.* (California: Celestial Arts, 1992).
[209]   Boutenko, Victoria, *Green for Life*, p. 63, citing: Minocha Anil M.D., Carrol David. *Natural Stomach Care: Treating and Preventing Digestive Disorders with the Best of Eastern and Western Healing Therapies*, (New York: Penguin Group, 2003).
[210]   Boutenko, Victoria, *Green for Life*, p. 62.
[211]   Boutenko, Victoria, *Green for Life*, (Raw Family Publishing, 2005), p. 66, citing: Stiteler L. Ac., O.M.D., N.M.D., *A Closer Look at Hypochlorhydria*. Stephen, Hom. California: The Institute of Bioterrain sciences, 2003. Accessible at: www.csupomona.edu
[212]   Boutenko, Victoria, *Green for Life*, p. 67, citing: Baroody, Dr. Theodore A., Jr. *Alkalize or Die.* (North Carolina: Eclectic Press, 1991).
[213]   Boutenko, Victoria, *Green for Life*, (Raw Family Publishing, Oregon, 2005), p. 74.

[214] Boutenko, Victoria, *Green for Life*, p. 76.

[215] The Raw Family website 2008-2010, www.rawfamily.com

[216] The Renegade Health Show episode #534, Top 10 Smoothie Ingredients Right Now.

[217] Wandling, Julie, *Thank God for Raw Recipes for Health*, (Healthy 4 Him Publishing, Akron, Ohio, 2002), p. 134.

[218] Holdstock, Sharon, *Shazzie's Detox Delights*, (Rawcreation, UK, 2001), p. 8-9.

[219] Kenney, Matthew; *Everyday Raw*, (Gibbs Smith, Publisher, Layton, Utah, 2008), p. 22, 30.

[220] Safron, Jeremy A., Underkoffler, Renee, *The Raw Truth the Art of Loving Foods*, (Raw Truth Press, Paia, HI, cir. 2004), p. 59, 60, 62.

[221] Shannon, Nomi, *The Raw Gourmet*, (Alive Books, Vancouver, Canada, 2001), p. 31.

[222] Cohen, Alissa, *Living on Live Food*, (Cohen Pub. Co., Kittery, ME, 2006), p. 538, 540, 541.

[223] Clement, Anna Maria, and Kelly Serbonich, *Healthful Cuisine,* (Healthful Communications, Juno Beach, FL, 2007), p. 20, 64-65.

[224] Rhio, Hooked on Raw (Beso Entertainment, P.O. Box 2040, Canal Street Station, New York, NY, 2000), pp. 192, 193, 194.

[225] Cousens, Gabriel, *Rainbow Green Live-Food Cuisine*, (North Atlantic Books, Berkeley, CA, 2003), pp. 292 293, 296.

Notes

[226] Kalechofsky, Roberta, *Judaism and Animal Rights*, (Micah Pub. Marblehead, MA., 2002) Rabbi Noach Valley, p. 201.

[227] Schwartz, Richard, Ph.D., *Vegetarianism and the Jewish Dietary Laws*, p. 4, The Schwartz Collection... (on his website).

[228] (Lev 10:10; 11:47; 20:25; Ezek 22:26)

[229] cleanness (Lev 15:13; 22:4); to cleanse (Lev 16:30; Num 8:6); to cleanse oneself (Num 8:7; Josh 22:17); purifying (Lev 12:4); cleansing (Lev 13:7: Num 6:9); clean (Gen 7:2; Lev 11:47)

[230] (Lev 14:52; Num 19:19; Ezek 43:20), and to cleanse oneself (Num 19:12-13, 20).

[231] (Job 15:14; 25:4; 33:9; Ps 73;13; Isa 1:16)

[232] (Is 35:8; 52:1; Ezek 39:24; Rev 21:27), or is... opposed to God (Zech 13:2; Mk 1:23; Lk 4:33; Ac 5:16), and ...abomination to Yahweh (Lev 7:21; 11:10; Deut 17:1).

[233] Schwartz, *Judaism and Vegetarianism*, p. 121, citing: Rabbi J. David Bleich, "Vegetarianism and Judaism," *Tradition*, Vol. 23, No. 1 (summer, 1987).

[234] Dionysius the Areopagite, *The Divine Names and Mystical Theology*, trans by C.E. Rolt, (SPCK, Holy Trinity Church, London, 1979), p. 55.

[235] Russell, Rex, M.D., *What the Bible Says About Healthy Living*, on the page 150. David Macht, M.D., "An Experimental Pharmacological Appreciation of Leviticus XI and Deuteronomy XIV," *Bulletin of Historical Medicine*, Johns Hopkins University, 47:1 (April 1953): pp. 444-450.

[236] Russell, Rex, M.D., *What the Bible Says About Healthy Living*, p. 150. Citing: David Macht, M.D., "An Experimental Pharmacological Appreciation of Leviticus XI and Deuteronomy XIV," *Bulletin of Historical Medicine*, Johns Hopkins University, 47:1 (April 1953): pp. 444-450.

[237] Russell, Rex, M.D., *What the Bible Says About Healthy Living*, p. 150. Citing: David Macht, M.D., "An Experimental Pharmacological Appreciation of Leviticus XI and Deuteronomy XIV," *Bulletin of Historical Medicine*, Johns Hopkins University, 47:1 (April 1953): pp. 444-450.

[238] Stegemann, Hartmut, *The Library of Qumran, On the Essenes, Qumran, John the Baptist, and Jesus* (William B. Eerdman's Publishing Company, Grand Rapids, Michigan, (1993 German) 1998 English), 267.

[239] *Encyclopedia of the Dead Sea Scrolls*, Editors Schiffman, VanderKam, p. 813, citing: *Jewish Antiquities* 13.171-173.

[240] *Encyclopedia of the Dead Sea...*, p. 264, citing: *The Jewish War* 2.145.

[241] *Encyclopedia of the Dead Sea...*, p. 264, citing: *The Jewish War*

2.136.

242 *Encyclopedia of the Dead Sea Scrolls*, p. 264, citing: *Refutatio* 9.27.

243 *Encyclopedia of the Dead Sea Scrolls*, p. 266, citing: 1 QS iv.6-8; CD iii.20; see also *Rule of Blessings* (1Q28b) iv.24-26.

244 *Encyclopedia of the Dead Sea Scrolls*, p. 266, citing: 4Q521.

245 Kalechofsky, *Vegetarian Judaism*, (Micah Publications, Inc., N.H. 1998), p. 48.

246 Feeley-Harnik, Gillian, Smithsonian Institution Press, Washington, D.C., 1994, p. 105, citing: *Flaccus*, 95-6.

247 Feeley-Harnik, Gillian, p. 106, citing: *The Jewish War*, 2:152-53.

248 Ewing, Upton Clary, *The Prophet of the Dead Sea Scrolls* (Tree of Life Publications, Joshua Tree, CA, 1993; 1963), p. 85, citing: Josephus *Life*, 3.

249 Thiering, Barbara, "The Biblical Source of Qumran Asceticism", p. 431, University of Sydney, Sydney, Australia, *Journal of Biblica Literature* Thiering, vol. 93, 1974, pp. 429-444.

250 Thiering, Barbara, "The Biblical Source of Qumran Asceticism", p. 443, citing: *Ant.* 13.11,1; 311; 15.105; 337; 17.5,6; 346.

251 Cousens, Gabriel, MD, *Creating Peace by Being Peace, p. 6.*

252 Ewing, *The Prophet of the Dead Sea Scrolls*, p. 122-123.

253 Ewing, *The Prophet of the Dead Sea Scrolls*, p. 122-123.

254 Rabbi Gabriel Cousens, *Modern Essenes A Brief Synopsis*, a handout (Monday July 2, 2012) at the Tree of Life conference for the Essene Gathering.

255 Pope Benedict XVI (Joseph Ratzinger), *Jesus of Nazareth, Holy Week: From the Entrance into Jerusalem to the Resurrection*, (Ignatius Press, San Francisco, 2011, Hardbound edition Doubleday Publishing), p. 106, 110, 111.

256 Pope Benedict XVI, *Jesus of Nazareth*, p. 224-225, citing: the French exegete Henri Cazelles, drawing on studies by J. Collson, J. Winandy, and M.E. Boismard. Cazelles, *"Johannes"* p. 481, pp. 480, 481.

257 Rabbi Gabriel Cousens, *Modern Essenes, A Brief Synopsis*, a handout (Monday July 2, 2012) at the Tree of Life conference for the Essene Gathering.

258 Rabbi Gabriel Cousens, *Modern Essenes, A Brief Synopsis*, a handout (Monday July 2, 2012) at the Tree of Life conference for the Essene Gathering.

259 McGowan, Andrew, *Ascetic Eucharists, Food and Drink in Early Christian Ritual Meals,* (Clarendon Press Oxford, New York, 1999), p. 149.

260 Joseph Cardinal Ratzinger released a document (Rome, the feast of the Ascension 2001) by the Pontifical Biblical Commission: *The Jewish People and Their Sacred Scriptures in the Christian Bible*, it speaks several times of the Essenes.

261 Joseph Cardinal Ratzinger released a document (Rome, the feast of the Ascension 2001) by the Pontifical Biblical Commission: *The Jewish*

People and Their Sacred Scriptures in the Christian Bible, it speaks several times of the Essenes.

262 Pope Benedict XVI (Joseph Ratzinger) *Jesus of Nazareth, from the Baptism in the Jordan to the Transfiguration*, (Ignatius Press, San Francisco, 2007, Hardbound edition Doubleday Publishing).

263 Pope Benedict XVI, *Jesus of Nazareth,* p. 13, 14.

264 Brown, Raphael, *The Life of Mary as Seen by the Mystics*, Tan Books and Publishers, Rockford, IL, 1951, reprinted 1991).

265 Brown, Raphael, *The Life of Mary as Seen by the Mystics*, p. 96.

266 Pope Benedict XVI (Joseph Ratzinger) *Jesus of Nazareth, from the Baptism in the Jordan to the Transfiguration*, (Ignatius Press, San Francisco, 2007, Hardbound edition Doubleday Publishing).

267 Pope Benedict XVI, *Jesus of Nazareth,* p. 13, 14.

268 Kalechofsky, *Judaism and Animal Rights*, p. 150-51, citing: Louis A. Berman, *The Dietary Laws as Atonements for Flesh-eating.*

269 Kalechofsky, *Judaism and Animal..*, p. 151, citing: Baba Batra 60b.

270 See Jewish Vegetarian Society or Professor Kalechofsky, PhD writings on Jewish vegetarianism.

271 *Encyclopedia of the Early Church*, Institutum Patristicum Augustinianum, (Oxford University Press, Inc., New York, N.Y., 1992).

272 *Encyclopedia of the Early Church*, citing: Iren., *Haer.* I 2,1 ; Tertull., *Ieiun.* 15, 1; Epiph., *Haer.* 30,18ff. and 47,1; Aug., *Haer.* 25.46.70.

273 Ewing, *The Prophet of the Dead Sea Scrolls*, p. 145, citing: *Hastings Encyclopedia on Religion and Ethics* (V.5, p. 143), Charles Scribner's, Sons, N.Y.

274 Ewing, *The Prophet of the Dead Sea Scrolls*, p. 145, citing: Teicher, J.L., *Journal of Jewish Studies*, 1951.

275 As explained in *A Critical Investigation of Epiphanius' Knowledge of the Ebionites: A Translation and Critical Discussion of "Panarion,"* by Glen Alan Kochit.

276 Cousens, Gabriel, *Conscious Eating*, p. 381.

277 *Encyclopedia of the Dead Sea Scrolls*, Editors Schiffman, VanderKam, p. 248, citing: *Adversus omnes Haereses* 1.28.

278 *Encyclopedia of the Early Church*, Institutum Patristicum Augustinianum, Oxford University Press, Inc., New York, N.Y., 1992.

279 *Encyclopedia of the Early Church*, citing: Hermas, *Past., Sim.* V 1,5; cf. Emped. fr B144.

280 *Encyclopedia of the Early Church*, citing: *ibid.* V3, 7; cf. Cypr., *Or* 32-33

281 *Encyclopedia of the Early Church*, citing: Hermas, *Past., Sim* 3,9.

282 *Encyclopedia of the Early Church*, citing: Clem. Al., *Paed.* II, 1, 1 ff.; Tertull., *Cult. fem* II 9.7; Orig., *In Jer.* 20,7; Euseb., *HE* V 3,2 and d.e.3, 5; Jerome, Jov. 5,18.

283 *Encyclopedia of the Early Church*, citing: Can. ap. 50 and 52.

284 *Encyclopedia of the Early Church*, citing: Iren., *Haer.* I 2,1 ; Tertull., *Ieiun.* 15, 1; Epiph., *Haer.* 30,18ff. and 47,1; Aug., *Haer.* 25.46.70.

[285] *Encyclopedia of the Early Church*, citing: *Ps Clem. rec.* VII 6,4; cf. Greg. Naz., *Or.* 14,4.

[286] Reference to Lawrence E. Frizzell, *Marian Studies*, XLVI (1995), p. 27-32; citing, see Mary Douglas in an appendix to Jacob Neusner, *The Idea of Purity in Judaism* (Leiden: E.J. Brill, 1973, 137-142.)

[287] Alonso, Joaquim, Maria; Ribeiro, Abilio Pina, *Fatima Message and Consecration*, (Consolata Missions Pub., Fatima, 1984, 1998), p. 61

[288] Alonso, Joaquim, Maria; Ribeiro, Abilio Pina, *Fatima Message and Consecration*, p. 58.

[289] Laurentin, Fr. Rene, *The Meaning of Consecration Today a Marian Model for a Secularized Age*, (Ignatius Press, San Francisco, 1992, French 1991), p. 35, 36.

[290] Laurentin, *The Meaning of Consecration Today*, p. 36.

[291] Laurentin, *The Meaning of Consecration Today*, p. 41, 42. Citing St. Augustine ...ipse homo, Dei nomine consecratus et Deo devotus, inquantum mundo moritur ut Deo vivat, sacrificium est" (De civitate Dei, liber 10 et 6, PL 41, 283).

[292] Cizik, Ladis, J., Fr., "Our Lady Keeps Her Promise," *Soul*, Jan.-Feb. 2001, p. 11.

[293] Ibid, Haffert, John, *God's Final Effort*, p. 74-75.

Notes

www.ingramcontent.com/pod-product-compliance
Lightning Source LLC
Chambersburg PA
CBHW030320290526
45785CB00001B/449